Fluids & Electrolytes

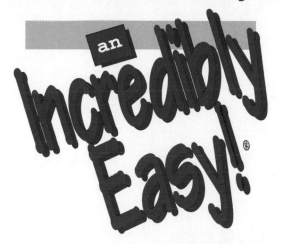

an Incredibly Easy!®

Pocket Guide

D0067222

Fluids & Electrolytes

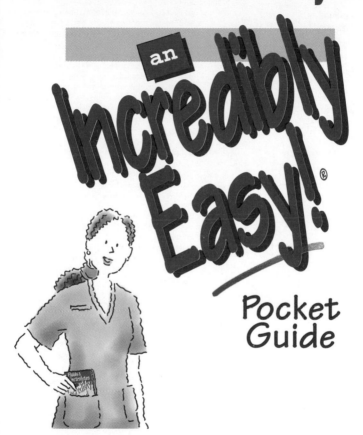

an *Incredibly Easy!*®

Pocket
Guide

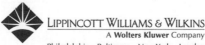

LIPPINCOTT WILLIAMS & WILKINS
A **Wolters Kluwer** Company

Philadelphia • Baltimore • New York • London
Buenos Aires • Hong Kong • Sydney • Tokyo

Staff

Executive Publisher
Judith A. Schilling McCann, RN, MSN

Editorial Director
David Moreau

Clinical Director
Joan M. Robinson, RN, MSN

Senior Art Director
Arlene Putterman

Art Director
Mary Ludwicki

Editorial Project Manager
Coleen M.F. Stern

Clinical Project Manager
Beverly Ann Tscheschlog, RN, BS

Editor
Amanda Bradford Cortright

Clinical Editor
Anita Lockhart, RN, C, MSN

Copy Editors
Kimberly Bilotta (supervisor),
Dorothy P. Terry, Pamela Wingrod

Designer
Lynn Foulk

Illustrator
Bot Roda

Digital Composition Services
Diane Paluba (manager), Joyce Rossi Biletz

Manufacturing
Patricia K. Dorshaw (director),
Beth J. Welsh

Editorial Assistants
Megan L. Aldinger, Karen J. Kirk,
Linda K. Ruhf

Indexer
Karen C. Comerford

F&EIEPG010705 — 031206

Library of Congress Cataloging-in-Publication Data
Fluids & electrolytes : an incredibly easy pocket guide.
    p. ; cm.
    Includes bibliographical references and index.
    1. Water-electrolyte imbalances — Handbooks, manuals, etc. 2. Water-electrolyte balance (Physiology) — Handbooks, manuals, etc. 3. Body fluid disorders — Handbooks, manuals, etc. 4. Acid-base imbalances — Handbooks, manuals, etc. I. Lippincott Williams & Wilkins. II. Title: Fluids and electrolytes. [DNLM: 1. Water-Electrolyte Imbalance — Handbooks. 2. Water-Electrolyte Balance — Handbooks. WD 200.1 F6462 2006]
    RC630.F5883 2006
    616.3'992 — dc22
    ISBN13 978-1-58255-433-4
    ISBN10 1-58255-433-1 (alk. paper)   2005006552

Contents

Contributors and consultants

Cheryl L. Brady, RN, MSN
Adjunct Faculty
Kent State University
East Liverpool, Ohio

Shari Regina Cammon, RN, MSN, CCRN
Clinical Risk Management and Safety
  Surveillance Associate
Merck & Co., Inc.
West Point, Pa.

Helen Fu, RN, MSN, FNP
Family Nurse Practitioner
Soteria Family Health Center
Plymouth, Minn.

Margaret M. Gingrich, RN, MSN
Associate Professor
Harrisburg (Pa.) Area Community College

David J. Hartman, RN, MSN, CRNP
Nurse Practitioner
University of Pennsylvania Health System
Philadelphia

Dawna Martich, RN, MSN
Clinical Trainer
American Healthways
Pittsburgh

Valerie Mignatti, RN, BSN
Cardiovascular Clinical Nurse
University of Pennsylvania Medical Center
Philadelphia

Sharon D. O'Kelley, RN, ADN, OCN
Clinical Nurse III
Duke University Hospital
Durham, N.C.

Sherry A. Parmenter, RD, LD
Clinical Dietitian
Fairfield Medical Center
Lancaster, Ohio

Abby Plambeck, RN, BSN
Consultant
Milwaukee

Theresa Pulvano, RN, BSN
Practical Nursing Instructor
Ocean County Votechnical School
Lakehurst, N.J.

Monica Narvaez Ramirez, RN, MSN
Instructor
University of the Incarnate Word
School of Nursing & Health Professions
San Antonio, Tex.

Patricia Weiskittel, RN, MSN, APRN,BC, CNN
Primary Care Nurse Practitioner
Internal Medicine
Veterans Administration Hospital
Cincinnati

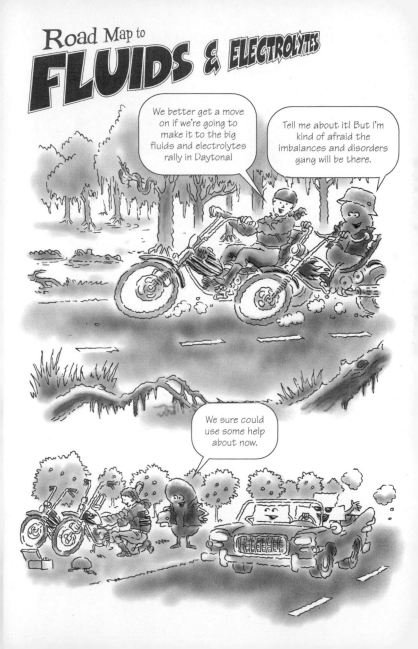

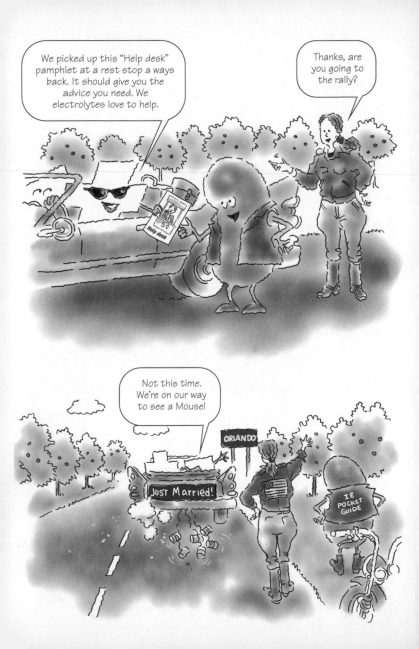

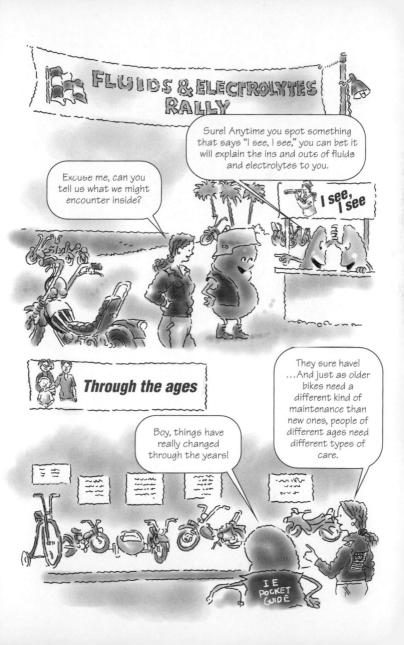

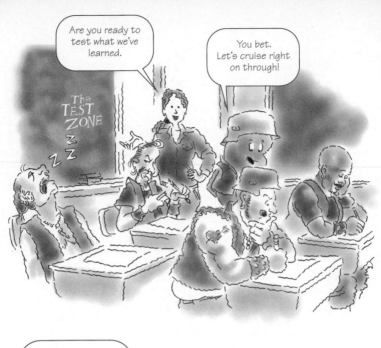
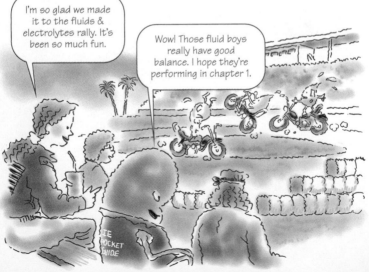

Balancing basics

1

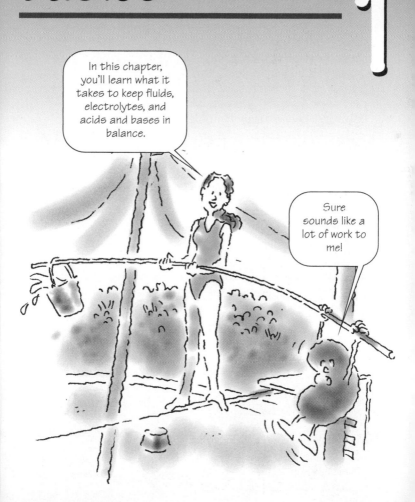

Fluid balance

Key facts

- Nearly all major organs in the body work together to maintain a balance of daily fluid gains and losses.
- Insensible fluid losses occur through the skin and lungs; they're called insensible because they can't be seen or measured.
- Sensible fluid losses occur through urination, defecation, and wounds; they're called sensible because they can be perceived or measured.

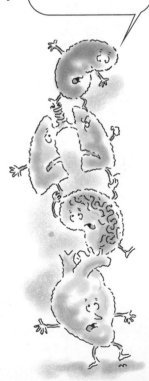

Major organs — including me — work together to maintain fluid balance.

Sites involved in fluid loss

Each day, the body gains and loses fluid through several different processes. Gastric, intestinal, pancreatic, and biliary secretions are almost completely reabsorbed and aren't usually counted in daily fluid losses and gains.

Daily total intake 2,600 ml
- Liquids 1,500 ml
- Solid foods 800 ml
- Water of oxidation 300 ml

Daily total output 2,600 ml
- Skin 600 ml
- Lungs 400 ml
- Kidneys (urine) 1,500 ml
- Intestines (feces) 100 ml

- The body holds intracellular fluid inside the cells (in the intracellular compartment) and outside the cells (in the extracellular compartment).
- To maintain balance, fluid distribution between the intracellular and extracellular compartments must remain constant.
- Extracellular fluid includes interstitial fluid, which surrounds the cells, and intravascular fluid (plasma), which is the liquid portion of blood.

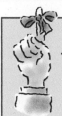

Memory jogger
To help you remember which fluid belongs in which compartment, keep in mind that **inter** means between (as in **inter**val — between two events) and **intra** means within or inside (as in **intra**venous — inside a vein).

Fluid types

- Body fluids may appear as isotonic, hypotonic, or hypertonic solutions.
- An isotonic solution has the same solute concentration as another solution.

Fluid compartments

The primary fluid compartments in the body are intracellular and extracellular. Extracellular is further divided into interstitial and intravascular. Capillary walls and cell membranes separate intracellular fluids from extracellular fluids.

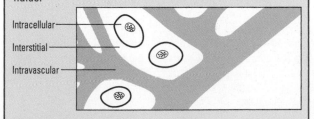

Intracellular
Interstitial
Intravascular

- Fluid doesn't shift between isotonic solutions because they're equally concentrated and already in balance.
- A hypotonic solution has a lower solute concentration than another solution.
- When a less concentrated (hypotonic) solution is placed next to a more concentrated (hypertonic) solution, fluid shifts from the hypotonic solution into the more concentrated compartment to equalize the concentrations.

Body fluids can be isotonic, hypotonic, or hypertonic solutions.

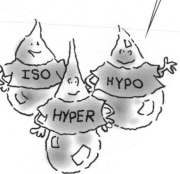

Through the ages

Fluid distribution and age

The risk of suffering a fluid imbalance increases with age because skeletal muscle mass declines and the proportion of fat within the body increases. After age 60, water content drops to about 45%.

Likewise, the distribution of fluid within the body changes with age. For example, infants store a greater percentage of body water in the interstitial spaces than adults. About 15% of a typical young adult's total body weight is made up of interstitial fluid. That percentage progressively decreases with age.

About 5% of the body's total fluid volume is made up of plasma. Plasma volume remains stable throughout life.

I see, I see

Understanding types of fluids

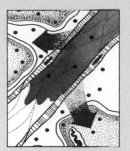

Hypotonic fluids
The solute concentration of a hypotonic solution is less than that of serum. Therefore, it shifts out of the intravascular compartment after administration.

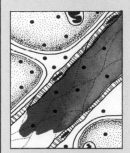

Isotonic fluids
The solute concentration of an isotonic solution is about equal to that of serum. Therefore, it stays in the intravascular space after administration.

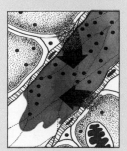

Hypertonic fluids
The solute concentration of a hypertonic solution is higher than that of serum. Therefore, it draws fluid into the intravascular space after administration.

- A hypertonic solution has a higher solute concentration than another solution.
- Although a hypertonic solution has more solutes than an adjacent solution, it has less fluid.

Fluid movement

- Fluids and solutes constantly shift within the body to maintain homeostasis.
- Solutes move through intracellular, interstitial, and intravascular compartments by crossing semipermeable membranes.
- Movement occurs through cells and capillaries.

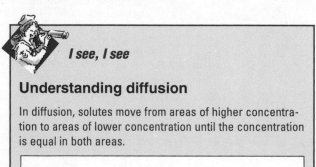

I see, I see

Understanding diffusion

In diffusion, solutes move from areas of higher concentration to areas of lower concentration until the concentration is equal in both areas.

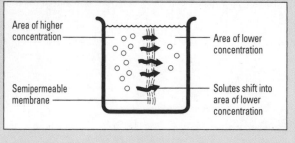

Area of higher concentration

Area of lower concentration

Semipermeable membrane

Solutes shift into area of lower concentration

Movement through cells

- In diffusion, solutes move from an area of higher concentration to an area of lower concentration. This requires no energy.
- In active transport, solutes move from an area of lower concentration to an area of higher concentration. This requires energy.
- In osmosis, fluid moves passively from an area with more fluid and fewer solutes to an area with less fluid and more solutes.

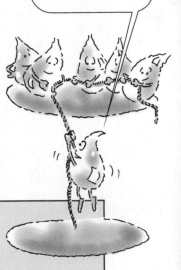

Boy, active transport takes a lot of energy. I need to get to higher ground!

I see, I see

Understanding active transport

During active transport, energy from a molecule called adenosine triphosphate (ATP) moves solutes from an area of lower concentration to an area of higher concentration.

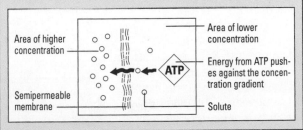

Area of higher concentration

Semipermeable membrane

Area of lower concentration

Energy from ATP pushes against the concentration gradient

Solute

ATP

I see, I see

Understanding osmosis

In osmosis, fluid moves passively from areas with more fluid (and fewer solutes) to areas with less fluid (and more solutes). Remember, in osmosis fluid moves, whereas in diffusion, solutes move.

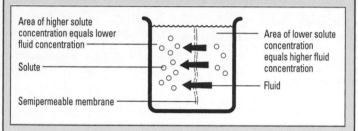

Area of higher solute concentration equals lower fluid concentration

Solute

Semipermeable membrane

Area of lower solute concentration equals higher fluid concentration

Fluid

Movement through capillaries

- Capillaries have walls thin enough to let solutes pass through.
- Fluids and solutes move through capillary walls to help maintain fluid balance.
- Hydrostatic pressure (the pressure of blood pushing against capillary walls) forces fluid and solutes through the walls.
- When the hydrostatic pressure inside a capillary is greater than the pressure in the surrounding interstitial space, fluids and solutes inside the capillary are forced into the interstitial space.
- When the pressure inside a capillary is less than the pressure outside it, fluids and solutes move back into the capillary.

To maintain balance, I move through capillary walls.

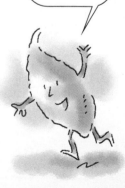

Fluid movement through the capillaries

When fluid-pushing, or *hydrostatic pressure,* builds inside a capillary, it forces fluids and solutes out through the capillary walls into the interstitial fluid, as shown below.

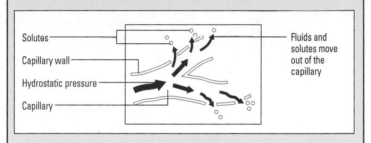

- Reabsorption prevents an excessive amount of fluid from leaving the capillaries.
- Within the capillaries, albumin acts like a water magnet to attract and hold water inside the vessel.
- The pulling force of albumin is known as the plasma colloid osmotic pressure.
- As long as hydrostatic pressure exceeds plasma colloid osmotic pressure, water and solutes can leave the capillaries and enter the interstitial fluid.
- When hydrostatic pressure falls below plasma colloid osmotic pressure, water and solutes return to the capillaries.

It's plasma colloid osmotic pressure, Daddy-O.

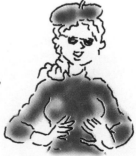

Maintaining fluid balance

- The kidneys and various hormones and mechanisms work together to maintain fluid balance.
- A problem in any of these can cause a fluid imbalance.

Kidneys

- In the kidneys, nephrons filter about 180 L of blood daily; this amount is the glomerular filtration rate.
- Nephrons produce 1 to 2 L of urine daily.
- The kidneys conserve water or excrete excess fluid to maintain balance.
- The minimum excretion rate varies with age.

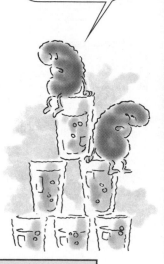

Good thing we conserve water when we need to, huh?

Through the ages

The higher the rate, the greater the waste

Infants and young children excrete urine at a higher rate than adults because they have higher metabolic rates. In addition, until about age 2, their kidneys are less efficient than those of an adult.

I see, I see

How antidiuretic hormone works

ADH regulates fluid balance through a series of steps, which are outlined below.

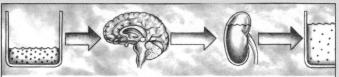

| The hypothalamus senses low blood volume and increased serum osmolality and signals the pituitary gland. | The pituitary gland secretes ADH into the bloodstream. | ADH causes the kidneys to retain water. | Water retention boosts blood volume and decreases serum osmolality. |

Antidiuretic hormone

- Antidiuretic hormone (ADH), or *vasopressin*, regulates fluid balance.
- ADH restores blood volume by reducing diuresis and increasing water retention.

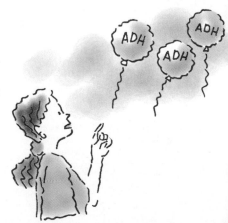

Renin-angiotensin-aldosterone system

- This mechanism helps maintain a balance of sodium and water and a healthy blood volume and pressure.
- When the fluid or sodium level falls, juxtaglomerular cells secrete renin, which stimulates angiotensin II production.
- Angiotensin II causes vasoconstriction and stimulates aldosterone production.
- Aldosterone causes sodium and water retention, leading to increased fluid volume and sodium levels.
- When blood pressure returns to normal, the body halts the release of renin, which stops this system.

I see, I see

How aldosterone works

Aldosterone, produced as a result of the renin-angiotensin mechanism, acts to regulate fluid volume, as described below.

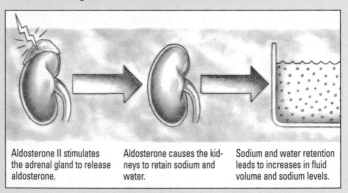

| Aldosterone II stimulates the adrenal gland to release aldosterone. | Aldosterone causes the kidneys to retain sodium and water. | Sodium and water retention leads to increases in fluid volume and sodium levels. |

Atrial natriuretic peptide
- Atrial natriuretic peptide (ANP) is a cardiac hormone.
- The actions of ANP oppose those of the renin-angiotensin-aldosterone system.
- ANP decreases blood pressure and reduces intravascular blood volume.
- Atrial stretching increases the amount of ANP released.

Thirst mechanism
- Thirst results from even small losses of fluid.
- When oral mucous membranes become dry, they stimulate the thirst center in the hypothalamus.

I see, I see

How atrial natriuretic peptide works

When blood volume and blood pressure rise and begin to stretch the atria, the heart's ANP shuts off the renin-angiotensin-aldosterone system, which stabilizes blood volume and blood pressure.

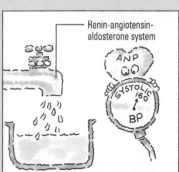
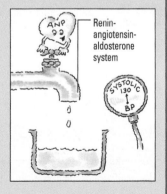

Electrolyte balance

Key facts

- Electrolytes work with fluids to maintain health and well-being.
- Electrolytes are substances that, when in a solution, separate into electrically charged particles called ions.
- Anions are electrolytes that produce a negative charge; cations are electrolytes that generate a positive charge.
- Extracellular electrolytes exert their effects outside the cells.
- Sodium and chloride are the major electrolytes in extracellular fluid; calcium and bicarbonate are also extracellular electrolytes.
- Intracellular electrolytes work inside the cells.
- Potassium, phosphate, and magnesium are the most plentiful intracellular electrolytes.

Organs and glands in electrolyte balance

- Lungs and liver—regulate sodium and water balance and blood pressure

Through the ages

Immature kidneys

The immature kidneys of an infant can't concentrate urine or reabsorb electrolytes as efficiently as an adult's kidneys, so the infant is at a higher risk for electrolyte imbalances.

Older adults are also at risk for electrolyte imbalances. Their kidneys have fewer functional nephrons, a decreased glomerular filtration rate, and a diminished ability to concentrate urine.

- Heart—secretes ANP, causing sodium excretion
- Sweat glands—excrete sodium, potassium, chloride, and water through sweat
- GI tract—absorbs and excretes fluids and electrolytes
- Parathyroid glands—secrete parathyroid hormone, which draws calcium into the blood and helps move phosphorus to the kidneys for excretion
- Thyroid gland—secretes calcitonin, which prevents calcium release from the bone

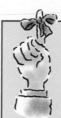

Memory Jogger

To remind yourself about the difference between anions and cations, remember that the *T* in "cation" looks like the positive symbol "+".

Looking on the plus and minus sides

Electrolytes can be either anions or cations. Here's a list of anions (the negative charges) and cations (the positive charges).

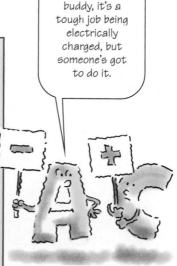

Well, old buddy, it's a tough job being electrically charged, but someone's got to do it.

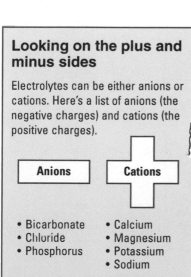

Anions	Cations
• Bicarbonate	• Calcium
• Chloride	• Magnesium
• Phosphorus	• Potassium
	• Sodium

Major electrolytes
Electrolytes can be either extracellular or intracellular.

Extracellular electrolytes
• Sodium — helps nerve cells and muscle cells interact
• Chloride — maintains osmotic pressure and helps gastric mucosal cells produce hydrochloric acid
• Calcium — stabilizes cell membranes and reduces permeability, transmits nerve impulses, contracts muscles, coagulates blood, and forms bones and teeth
• Bicarbonate — plays a role in acid-base balance

Intracellular electrolytes
• Potassium — responsible for cell excitability, nerve impulse conduction, resting membrane potential, muscle contraction, myocardial membrane responsiveness, and intracellular osmolality
• Phosphate — responsible for energy metabolism
• Magnesium — responsible for enzyme reactions, neuromuscular contractions, normal functioning of nervous and cardiovascular systems, protein synthesis, and sodium and potassium ion transportation

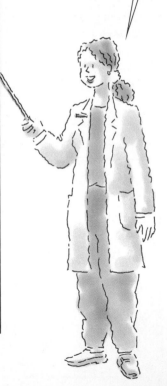

Sodium, chloride, potassium, phosphate — who do we appreciate?

Normal electrolyte levels

To maintain homeostasis, the body keeps electrolytes within a normal range, as shown below. All normal electrolyte levels are measured in serum.

Electrolyte	Normal levels
Sodium	135 to 145 mEq/L (SI, 135 to 145 mmol/L)
Potassium	3.5 to 5 mEq/L (SI, 3.5 to 5 mmol/L)
Calcium, total	8.2 to 10.2 mg/dl (SI, 2.05 to 2.54 mmol/L)
Calcium, ionized	4.65 to 5.28 mg/dl (SI, 1.1 to 1.25 mmol/L)
Phosphates	2.7 to 4.5 mg/dl (SI, 0.87 to 1.45 mmol/L)
Magnesium	1.3 to 2.1 mEq/L (SI, 1.3 to 2.1 mmol/L)
Chloride	100 to 108 mEq/L (SI, 100 to 108 mmol/L)

Factors affecting electrolyte balance

- Fluid intake and output
- Acid-base balance
- Hormone secretion
- Normal cell functioning

Electrolyte levels

- Only extracellular (serum) electrolyte levels are measured.
- Electrolyte levels are reported in milliequivalents per liter (mEq/L [SI, mmol/L]) or milligrams per deciliter (mg/dl [SI, mmol/L]), a measure of the ions' chemical activity.

Acid-base balance

Key facts
- The chemical reactions that sustain life depend on a balance between acids and bases in the body.
- Acids consist of molecules that can give up hydrogen molecules to other molecules, as in solutions with pH levels less than 7 (SI, 7).
- Bases consist of molecules that can accept hydrogen molecules, as in solutions with pH levels greater than 7 (SI, 7).
- To assess acid-base balance, you must know the pH level of the blood.
- Normally, pH ranges from 7.35 to 7.45 (SI, 7.35 to 7.45), which is slightly alkaline.
- A pH level less than 7.35 (SI, 7.35) is abnormally acidic; a pH level greater than 7.45 (SI, 7.45) is abnormally alkaline.

Acid-base regulators
- When pH rises or falls, three systems work to create acid-base balance.
- Chemical buffers instantly combine with the offending acid or base, neutralizing harmful effects until other regulators take over.
- The respiratory system uses hypoventilation and hyperventilation to regulate acid excretion or retention within minutes of pH change.
- The kidneys excrete or retain more acids or bases as needed, restoring the normal balance within hours or days.

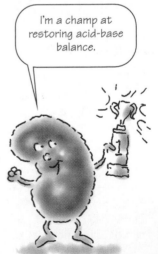

I'm a champ at restoring acid-base balance.

ABG analysis

- Arterial blood gas (ABG) analysis can help assess breathing effectiveness and acid-base balance.
- This test also helps monitor a patient's response to treatment.
- When interpreting ABG values, follow a consistent sequence to analyze the information.

Deviation from normal pH

- Compromises well-being, electrolyte balance, activity of critical enzymes, muscle contraction, and basic cellular function
- Is usually fatal if below 6.8 (SI, 6.8) or above 7.8 (SI, 7.8)
- Indicates alkalosis if above 7.45 (SI, 7.45)
- Indicates acidosis if below 7.35 (SI, 7.35)

Determine pH

- Check pH first because this figure forms the basis for understanding most other figures.
- If the pH level is abnormal, determine whether it reflects acidosis (less than 7.35 [SI, 7.35]) or alkalosis (greater than 7.45 [SI, 7.45]).
- Then figure out whether the cause is respiratory or metabolic.

Through the ages

Acid-base balance across the lifespan

The effectiveness of the systems that regulate acid-base balance varies with age; an infant's kidneys can't acidify urine as well as an adult's. The respiratory system of an older adult may be compromised and less able to regulate acid-base balance. In addition, because ammonia production decreases with age, the kidneys of an older adult can't handle excess acid as well as the kidneys of a younger adult.

Determine Paco₂

- Remember, the partial pressure of arterial carbon dioxide ($Paco_2$) value provides information about the respiratory component of acid-base balance.

- If the $Paco_2$ value is abnormal, determine whether it's low (less than 35 mm Hg [SI, 4.7 kPa]) or high (greater than 45 mm Hg [SI, 5.3 kPa]).
- Then determine whether the abnormal result corresponds with a change in pH.
- If pH is high, expect $Paco_2$ to be low (hypocapnia), indicating the problem is respiratory alkalosis.
- If pH is low, expect $Paco_2$ to be high (hypercapnia), indicating the problem is respiratory acidosis.

Watch the bicarbonate

- Examine the bicarbonate (HCO_3^-) value, which provides information about the metabolic aspect of acid-base balance.
- If the HCO_3^- value is abnormal, determine whether it's low (less than 22 mEq/L [SI, 22 mmol/L]) or high (greater than 25 mEq/L [SI, 25 mmol/L]).
- Then determine whether the abnormal result corresponds with a change in pH.

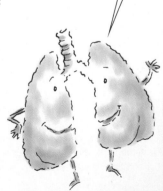

The $Paco_2$ value reflects the respiratory component of acid-base balance.

- If pH is high, expect HCO_3^- to be high, indicating the problem is metabolic alkalosis.
- If pH is low, expect HCO_3^- to be low, indicating the problem is metabolic acidosis.

Compensation can be either complete or partial.

Look for compensation

- Check for a change in the $Paco_2$ and HCO_3^- values. One value indicates the primary source of the pH change. The other indicates the body's effort to compensate for the disturbance.
- Consider whether compensation is complete or partial.
- Complete compensation occurs when the body compensates so effectively that pH falls within the normal range.
- Partial compensation occurs when pH remains outside the normal range.
- Compensation involves opposites. For example, if results indicate primary metabolic acidosis, compensation will take the form of respiratory alkalosis.

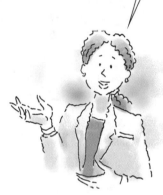

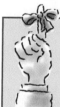

Memory jogger

Remember, HCO_3^- and pH increase or decrease together. When one rises or falls, so does the other.

Remember, $Paco_2$ and pH move in opposite directions. If $Paco_2$ rises, then pH falls and vice versa.

Determine Pao$_2$ and Sao$_2$

- Check the partial pressure of arterial oxygen (Pao$_2$) and arterial oxygen saturation (Sao$_2$) values, which provide information about the patient's oxygenation.

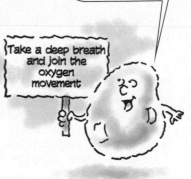

The Pao$_2$ and Sao$_2$ values give you information about your patient's oxygenation.

Take a deep breath and join the oxygen movement

- If the values are abnormal, determine whether they're high (Pao$_2$ greater than 100 mm Hg [SI, 13.3 kPa]) or low (Pao$_2$ less than 80 mm Hg [SI, 10.6 kPa] and Sao$_2$ less than 94% [SI, 0.94]).
- Consider the implications of your findings. Pao$_2$ reflects the body's ability to pick up oxygen from the lungs.
- A low Pao$_2$ value represents hypoxemia and can cause hyperventilation.
- The Pao$_2$ value also indicates when to make adjustments in the concentration of oxygen being given to a patient.

Avoid inaccurate ABG values

- To prevent inaccurate ABG values, be sure to use proper technique.
- Avoid delays in getting the sample to the laboratory.
- Don't draw blood for ABG analysis within 15 to 20 minutes of a procedure, such as suctioning or administering a respiratory treatment.
- Remove air bubbles from the syringe because they could affect the blood sample's oxygen level.
- Don't get venous blood in the syringe because it could alter the sample's carbon dioxide and oxygen levels and pH.

Fluid imbalances

2

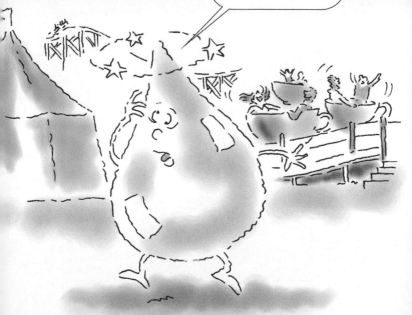

Chapter 2 takes a look at fluid volume and fluid imbalances. Talk about imbalance... whew!

A look at fluid volume

- Blood pressure is related to the amount of blood the heart pumps and the extent of vasoconstriction present.
- Fluid volume affects these elements, making blood pressure measurement key in assessing fluid status.
- Pulmonary artery pressure (PAP) and central venous pressure (CVP) also help assess fluid volume status.

> Measuring blood pressure is an important step in assessing fluid volume.

Cuff measurements

Key facts

- Direct and indirect blood pressure measurements are related to the amount of blood flowing through the patient's circulatory system.

A sizeable task

- Make sure the cuff is the correct size to avoid false readings.
- The bladder of the cuff should have a width of about 40% of the upper arm circumference.

In position

- Place the center of the cuff bladder directly over the median aspect of the arm.
- Palpate the brachial artery and place the bell of the stethoscope directly over this point.

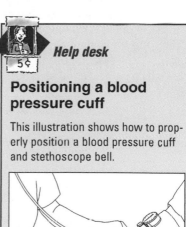

Help desk

Positioning a blood pressure cuff

This illustration shows how to properly position a blood pressure cuff and stethoscope bell.

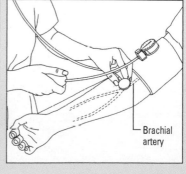

Brachial artery

It's automatic

- An automated blood pressure unit is designed to take readings repeatedly.
- It also computes and digitally records the readings.
- The monitor can be programmed to take readings as often as necessary.

Palpable pressure

- Palpable pressure estimates systolic blood pressure.
- It's used if there's difficulty hearing the patient's blood pressure, especially during hypotension.
- Place the cuff on the patient's arm — just like taking a blood pressure reading using a stethoscope.
- Palpate the brachial or radial pulse and then inflate the cuff until the pulse is no longer felt.
- Then, slowly deflate the cuff, noting when the pulse is felt again — the systolic blood pressure.
- Record a palpable pulse as "90/P." (The P stands for palpable.)

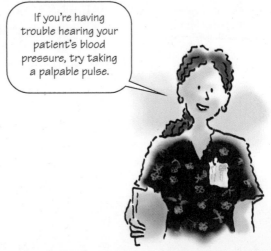

If you're having trouble hearing your patient's blood pressure, try taking a palpable pulse.

Help desk

Correcting problems of blood pressure measurement

Use this chart to figure out what to do for each possible cause of a false-high or false-low blood pressure reading.

Problem and possible cause	What to do
False-high reading	
Cuff too small	Make sure the cuff bladder is long enough to completely encircle the extremity.
Cuff wrapped too loosely, reducing its effective width	Tighten the cuff.
Slow cuff deflation, causing venous congestion in the arm or leg	Never deflate the cuff slower than 2 mm Hg/heartbeat.
Tilted mercury column	Read pressures with the mercury column vertical.
Poorly timed measurement (after the patient has eaten, ambulated, appeared anxious, or flexed his arm muscles)	Postpone blood pressure measurement, or help the patient relax before taking pressures.
Multiple attempts at reading blood pressure in the same arm, causing venous congestion	Don't measure blood pressure more than twice in the same arm; wait between attempts.

(continued)

Correcting problems of blood pressure measurement
(continued)

Problem and possible cause	What to do
False-low reading	
Incorrect position of the arm or leg	Make sure the arm or leg is level with the patient's heart.
Mercury column below eye level	Read mercury column at eye level.
Failure to notice auscultatory gap (sound fades out for 10 to 15 mm Hg, then returns)	Estimate systolic pressure using palpation before actually measuring it. Then check the palpable pressure against the measured pressure.
Inaudible or low-volume sounds	Before reinflating the cuff, instruct the patient to raise his arm or leg to decrease venous pressure and amplify low-volume sounds. After inflating the cuff, tell the patient to lower his arm or leg. Then deflate the cuff and listen. If you still fail to detect low-volume sounds, chart the palpable systolic pressure.

The Doppler difference

- A Doppler probe uses ultrasound waves directed at the blood vessel to detect blood flow.
- It's used if the patient's arm is swollen or pressure is so low that you can't feel the pulse.
- Record a Doppler reading as "90/D." (The D stands for Doppler.)

Help desk

How to take a Doppler blood pressure

When you can't hear or palpate a patient's blood pressure, try using a Doppler ultrasound device, as shown below.

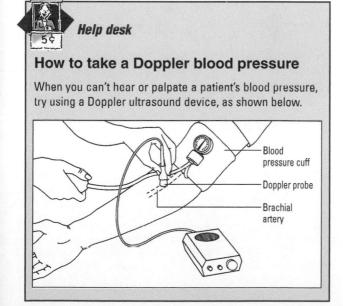

Blood pressure cuff

Doppler probe

Brachial artery

Direct measurements

Key facts

- A direct measurement is an invasive method of obtaining blood pressure readings.
- It uses an arterial catheter.
- It's used when highly accurate or frequent blood pressure measurements are required, as in severe fluid imbalances.

Arterial line

- An arterial line continually monitors blood pressure and can be used to sample arterial blood for blood gas analysis.
- It's inserted into the radial or brachial artery (or the femoral artery if needed).

Pulmonary artery catheter

- A pulmonary artery (PA) catheter directly measures other pressures.
- It's typically inserted into the subclavian vein or the internal jugular vein.
- The tip of the catheter rests in the pulmonary artery.

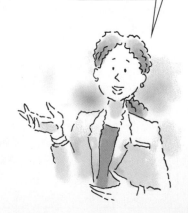

When frequent or highly accurate blood pressure measurements are needed, an arterial line gets the job done.

A clearer picture

- A PA catheter provides a clearer picture of the patient's fluid volume status than other measurements.
- It allows for measurement of PAP, pulmonary artery wedge pressure (PAWP), cardiac output, and CVP.
- Normal systolic PAP is 15 to 25 mm Hg.
- Systolic PAP reflects pressure from contraction of the right atrium.
- Normal diastolic PAP is 8 to 15 mm Hg.
- Diastolic PAP reflects the lowest pressure in the pulmonary vessels.
- Mean PAP is 10 to 20 mm Hg.

Central venous catheter

- A central venous catheter can measure CVP, another useful indication of a patient's fluid status.
- It measures the pressure of the blood in the central circulation.

A PA catheter or a central venous catheter can be used to measure fluid volume.

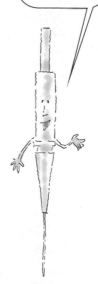

Help desk

Estimating CVP

To estimate a patient's CVP, follow these steps:

1. Place the patient at a 45- to 60-degree angle.

2. Use tangential lighting to observe the internal jugular vein.

3. Note the highest level of visible pulsation.

4. Locate the angle of Louis, or sternal notch, by palpating the point at which the clavicles join the sternum (the suprasternal notch).

5. Place two fingers on the patient's suprasternal notch and slide them down the sternum until they reach the bony protu-

berance known as the angle of Louis. The right atrium lies about 2″ (5 cm) below this point.

6. Measure the distance between the angle of Louis and the highest level of visible pulsation. Normally, this distance is less than 1⅛″ (3 cm).

7. Add 2″ to this figure to estimate the distance between the highest level of pulsation and the right atrium. A distance greater than 4″ (10 cm) may indicate elevated CVP.

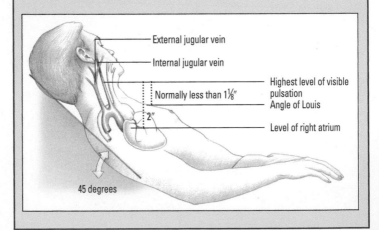

External jugular vein

Internal jugular vein

Normally less than 1⅛″

Highest level of visible pulsation

Angle of Louis

2″

Level of right atrium

45 degrees

A look at fluid imbalance

- When the body can't compensate for fluid deficits or excesses, an imbalance occurs.
- Fluid imbalances include dehydration, hypervolemia, hypovolemia, and water intoxication.
- Changes in fluid volume commonly affect blood pressure, which makes it a critical assessment.
- Changes in fluid volume may also affect PAP, CVP, PAWP, and cardiac output.

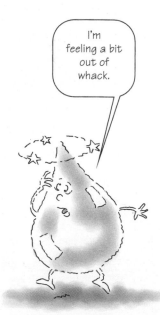

I'm feeling a bit out of whack.

Dehydration

Key facts

- The body constantly loses water, and a person responds by drinking fluids and consuming foods that contain water.
- If lost water isn't adequately replaced, the cells lose water, which can lead to dehydration.

I see, I see

What happens in dehydration

| Body loses fluid. |

▼

| Blood solute concentration (osmolality) increases. |

▼

| Serum sodium level rises. |

▼

| Water molecules shift out of cells into more concentrated blood. |

▼

| Water intake and retention aren't sufficient to restore fluid volume. |

▼

| Cells shrink as more fluid shifts out of them. |

▼

| Patient develops mental status changes, which may lead to seizures and coma. |

What causes it

- Diabetes insipidus
- Fever
- Diarrhea
- Renal failure
- Hyperglycemia

What to look for

- Irritability and confusion
- Dizziness
- Weakness
- Extreme thirst
- Fever
- Dry skin and mucous membranes
- Sunken eyeballs
- Poor skin turgor
- Decreased urine output
- Increased heart rate with decreased blood pressure

Through the ages

Different but the same

Elderly patients and very young patients are more susceptible to fluid and electrolyte imbalances. Despite the significant age difference, the contributing factors for these imbalances are the same in many cases:
- Inability to obtain fluid without help
- Inability to express feelings of thirst
- Inaccurate assessment of output; for example, if the patient must wear a diaper
- Loss of fluid through perspiration because of fever
- Loss of fluid through diarrhea and vomiting

What tests show

- Elevated hematocrit (HCT)
- Serum osmolality greater than 300 mOsm/kg (or 50 to 200 mOsm/kg in a patient with diabetes insipidus)
- Serum sodium level greater than 145 mEq/L (SI, 145 mmol/L)
- Urine specific gravity greater than 1.030 (or less than 1.005 in a patient with diabetes insipidus)

How it's treated

- Encourage the patient to drink salt-free oral fluids if tolerated.
- Begin emergency treatment if the patient displays impaired mental status, seizures, or coma.
- Administer I.V. fluids to a severely dehydrated patient using hypotonic, low-sodium solutions such as dextrose 5% in water.
- Replace lost fluids gradually over 48 hours.
- Assess for signs and symptoms of cerebral edema, which can result from I.V. solutions administered too rapidly.
- Administer vasopressin to a patient with diabetes insipidus if prescribed.
- Assess for complications of concentrated vascular volume, including thrombophlebitis and pulmonary emboli.
- Assess for diaphoresis, which can be a major source of water loss.
- Monitor the patient's sodium level, urine osmolality, and urine specific gravity.

> ### Signs and symptoms of cerebral edema
>
> - Headache
> - Confusion
> - Irritability
> - Lethargy
> - Nausea and vomiting
> - Widening pulse pressure
> - Decreasing pulse rate
> - Seizures

We need to replace those lost fluids.

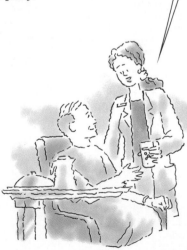

Hypervolemia

Key facts

- Hypervolemia is an excess of isotonic fluid (water and sodium) in the extracellular (interstitial or intravascular) compartment.
- This fluid imbalance usually doesn't affect osmolality because fluids and solutes are gained in equal proportions.
- With mild to moderate hypervolemia, a patient's weight may increase 5% to 10%; with severe hypervolemia, it may increase more than 10%.
- Elderly patients and patients with impaired renal or cardiovascular function are most susceptible to hypervolemia.

I see, I see

What happens in hypervolemia

Excess sodium or fluid is consumed or retained.

Fluid moves out of blood vessels into the interstitial space.

Extracellular fluid accumulates in the interstitial or intravascular compartment.

Edema develops in the lungs and other tissues.

What causes it

- Excess sodium or fluid intake
  - I.V. administration of normal saline or lactated Ringer's solution
  - Blood or plasma replacement
  - High intake of dietary sodium
- Fluid and sodium retention
  - Heart failure
  - Cirrhosis
  - Nephrotic syndrome
  - Corticosteroid use
  - Hyperaldosteronism
  - Low intake of dietary protein

Evaluating pitting edema

You can evaluate edema using a scale of +1 to +4. Press your fingertip firmly into the skin over a bony surface for a few seconds. Then note the depth of the imprint your finger leaves on the skin.

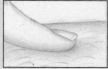 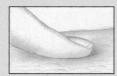 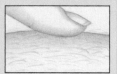

A slight imprint indicates +1 pitting edema.

A deep imprint, with the skin slow to return to its original contour, indicates +4 pitting edema.

When the skin resists pressure but appears distended, the condition is called brawny edema. In brawny edema, the skin swells so much that fluid can't be displaced.

How pulmonary edema develops

Excess fluid volume that lasts a long time can cause pulmonary edema. These illustrations show how that process occurs.

Normal

Normal pulmonary fluid movement depends on the equal force of two opposing pressures — hydrostatic pressure and plasma oncotic pressure from protein molecules in the blood.

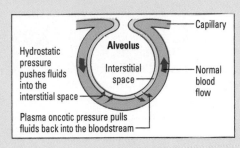

Congestion

Abnormally high pulmonary hydrostatic pressure (indicated by increased PAWP) forces fluid out of the capillaries and into the interstitial space, causing pulmonary congestion.

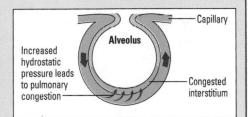

Edema

When the amount of interstitial fluid is excessive, fluid is forced into the alveoli; pulmonary edema results. Fluid fills the alveoli preventing gas exchange.

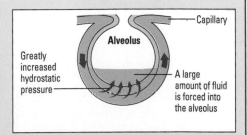

- Fluid shift into the intravascular space
  - Fluid movement after burn treatment
  - I.V. administration of hypertonic fluid
  - Use of albumin or other plasma proteins

What to look for
- Tachypnea and dyspnea
- Crackles
- Rapid, bounding pulse
- Hypertension (unless the heart is failing)
- Increased CVP, PAP, and PAWP
- Distended jugular and hand veins
- Acute weight gain
- Peripheral edema
- S_3 gallop
- Pulmonary edema (with prolonged hypervolemia)

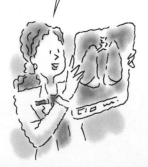

If you see pulmonary congestion on a chest X-ray, hypervolemia may be the cause.

What tests show
- Low HCT because of hemodilution
- Normal serum sodium level
- Lower serum potassium and blood urea nitrogen (BUN) levels because of hemodilution (or higher levels in a patient with renal failure or impaired renal perfusion)
- Low oxygen level
- Pulmonary congestion on chest X-rays

How it's treated
- Restrict the patient's sodium and fluid intake.
- Administer diuretics as prescribed.
- Provide oxygen therapy.
- Treat heart failure with digoxin and bed rest.
- Treat pulmonary edema with drugs that dilate blood vessels, such as morphine and nitroglycerin.
- If the patient has renal failure and diuretics aren't effective, provide hemodialysis or another form of dialysis.
- Assess for signs and symptoms of hypovolemia, which can result from overcorrection of hypervolemia.
- Monitor the results of arterial blood gas analysis to detect changes in oxygenation and acid-base balance.
- Monitor the patient's potassium level, which typically decreases with diuretic use and increases with renal failure.
- Assess for an S_3 heart sound that's heard when the ventricles are volume-overloaded.

Hypovolemia

Key facts

- Hypovolemia refers to an isotonic fluid loss — including the loss of fluids and solutes — from the extracellular space.
- If hypovolemia isn't detected early and treated, it may progress to hypovolemic shock.

I see, I see

What happens in hypovolemia with third-space shifting

> Capillary membrane permeability increases or plasma colloid osmotic pressure decreases.

⬇

> Fluid moves out of the intravascular space.

⬇

> Fluid shifts into the abdominal cavity, pleural cavity, or pericardial sac.

⬇

> Reduced fluid intake may exacerbate the fluid shift.

⬇

> Patient displays weight loss, mental status changes, and orthostatic hypotension.

What causes it

- Excessive fluid loss
  - Abdominal surgery
  - Diabetes mellitus (from polyuria)
  - Diarrhea
  - Excessive diuretic therapy
  - Excessive laxative use
  - Excessive sweating
  - Fever
  - Fistulas
  - Hemorrhage
  - Nasogastric (NG) tube drainage
  - Renal failure with polyuria
  - Vomiting
- Third-space shifting
  - Acute intestinal obstruction
  - Acute peritonitis
  - Burns (in the initial phase)
  - Crush injuries
  - Hip fracture
  - Hypoalbuminemia
  - Pleural effusion

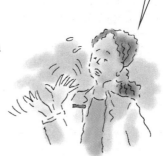

Excessive sweating is one of the many causes of hypovolemia.

What to look for

- Altered mental status
- Tachycardia
- Orthostatic hypotension followed by marked hypotension
- Decreased urine output (10 to 30 ml/hour)
- Weight loss
- Cool, pale skin over arms and legs
- Delayed capillary refill
- Thirst
- Flat jugular veins
- Decreased CVP

What tests show
- Decreased hemoglobin level and HCT, with hemorrhage
- Elevated BUN level
- Increased urine specific gravity, with the kidneys trying to conserve fluid
- Normal or high serum sodium level (greater than 145 mEq/L [SI, 145 mmol/L]), depending on the amount of fluid and sodium lost

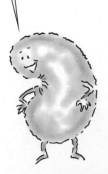

If tests indicate a patient's urine specific gravity has increased, it might mean I'm trying to conserve fluid because of hypovolemia.

How it's treated

- Replace lost fluids with isotonic solutions (fluids of the same concentration).
- Administer I.V. fluids in a fluid challenge, giving them in large amounts over a short time. Use short, large-bore catheters for rapid infusion.
- Provide numerous I.V. infusions for hypovolemic shock.
- Administer oxygen.
- Lower the head of the bed or elevate the foot of the bed to increase cerebral perfusion.
- Administer a vasopressor, such as dopamine, to raise the patient's blood pressure.
- Administer blood transfusions if the patient is hemorrhaging.
- Monitor hemodynamic values (CVP, PAP, PAWP, and cardiac output) to assess the patient's response to treatment.
- Monitor for signs and symptoms of fluid overload, such as crackles, which may result from aggressive fluid replacement.
- Closely monitor the patient's mental status and vital signs, staying alert for blood pressure changes and arrhythmias.

Hemodynamic values in hypovolemic shock

Hemodynamic monitoring helps in evaluating the patient's cardiovascular status in hypovolemic shock. Look for these values:

- CVP below the normal range of 5 to 10 cm H_2O
- PAP below the normal mean of 10 to 20 mm Hg
- PAWP below the normal mean of 6 to 12 mm Hg
- Cardiac output below the normal range of 8 L/minute.

Water intoxication

Key facts

- Water intoxication occurs when excess fluid moves from the extracellular space to the intracellular space.

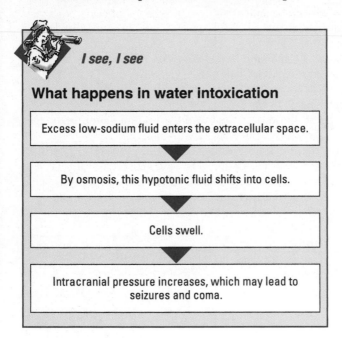

I see, I see

What happens in water intoxication

Excess low-sodium fluid enters the extracellular space.

By osmosis, this hypotonic fluid shifts into cells.

Cells swell.

Intracranial pressure increases, which may lead to seizures and coma.

What causes it

- Syndrome of inappropriate antidiuretic hormone secretion
- Rapid infusion of a hypotonic solution
- Excessive use of tap water as an NG tube irrigant or enema
- Psychogenic polydipsia

What to look for
- Increased intracranial pressure
- Muscle cramps and weakness
- Nausea and vomiting
- Headache
- Changes in personality, behavior, and level of consciousness
- Twitching
- Thirst
- Dyspnea on exertion
- Bradycardia and widened pulse pressure

What tests tell you
- Serum osmolality less than 280 mOsm/kg
- Serum sodium level less than 125 mEq/L (SI, 125 mmol/L)

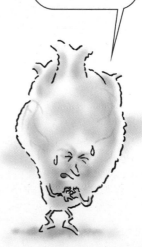

Bradycardia and widened pulse pressure are signs of water intoxication.

How it's treated

- Correct the underlying cause. For example, slow or temporarily discontinue a hypotonic solution infusion, or replace tap water with sterile water or a hypertonic solution for NG tube irrigation or enemas.
- Restrict oral and parenteral fluid intake and avoid the use of hypotonic I.V. solutions until the patient's serum sodium level rises.
- Administer a hypertonic I.V. solution slowly, using an infusion pump.
- Monitor the patient's neurologic status, staying alert for deterioration.
- Monitor the patient's serum sodium level.
- Institute seizure precautions as needed.

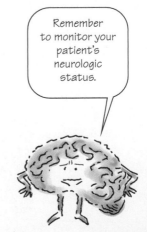

Remember to monitor your patient's neurologic status.

Electrolyte imbalances

3

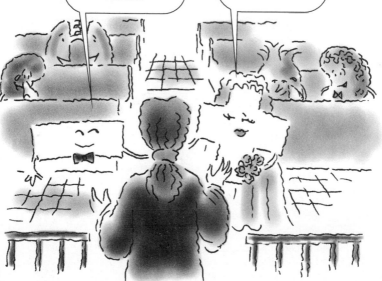

Hypernatremia

Key facts

- Hypernatremia is characterized by a serum sodium level greater than 145 mEq/L (SI, 145 mmol/L).
- In hypernatremia, the body has an excess of sodium relative to water.
- Severe hypernatremia can lead to seizures, coma, and permanent neurologic damage.

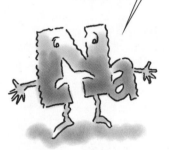

When the body has too much of me it's called hypernatremia.

I see, I see

What happens in hypernatremia

Sodium intake or water loss becomes excessive.

Serum osmolality increases.

Fluid moves by osmosis from inside of the cells to outside of the cells to balance intracellular and extracellular fluid levels.

Cells become dehydrated, causing neurologic impairment; extracellular fluid volume in vessels increases, causing hypervolemia.

What causes it

- Water deficit
  - Fever
  - Heat stroke
  - Pulmonary infections
  - Extensive burns
  - Severe diarrhea
  - Hyperosmolar hyperglycemic nonketotic syndrome
  - Urea diuresis
  - Diabetes insipidus
- Excess sodium intake
  - Overconsumption of dietary sodium
  - Use of certain drugs
  - Near drowning in salt water
  - Cushing's syndrome
  - Hyperaldosteronism

Drugs that can cause hypernatremia

- Antacids with sodium bicarbonate
- Antibiotics, such as ticarcillin disodium-clavulanate potassium
- Salt tablets
- Sodium bicarbonate injections such as those given during cardiac arrest
- I.V. sodium chloride preparations
- Sodium polystyrene sulfonate

What to look for

- Agitation and restlessness
- Confusion
- Flushed skin

Through the ages

Greater risk for hypernatremia

Infants and children are at greater risk for hypernatremia because they tend to lose more water as a result of diarrhea, vomiting, inadequate fluid intake, and fever.

- Intense thirst
- Lethargy
- Low-grade fever
- Signs and symptoms of hypervolemia (from sodium gain), such as bounding pulses, dyspnea, and hypertension
- Signs and symptoms of hypovolemia (from water loss), such as dry mucous membranes, oliguria, and orthostatic hypotension
- Twitching
- Weakness

What tests show

- Serum osmolality greater than 300 mOsm/kg
- Serum sodium level greater than 145 mEq/L (SI, 145 mmol/L)
- Urine specific gravity greater than 1.030 (or less than 1.005 in a patient with diabetes insipidus)

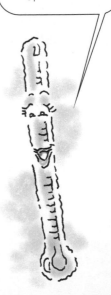

A low-grade fever is one of the signs of hypernatremia.

How it's treated

- Individualize treatment based on the cause of hypernatremia.
- Replace oral fluids gradually over 48 hours to avoid shifting water into brain cells. If too much water is replaced too quickly, water moves into brain cells and they swell, causing cerebral edema.
- Replace fluids with a salt-free I.V. solution such as dextrose 5% in water. Use an infusion pump to help prevent cerebral edema.
- Infuse half-normal saline solution to prevent hyponatremia and cerebral edema.
- Restrict the patient's sodium intake.
- Administer a diuretic along with oral or I.V. fluids.
- Frequently check the patient's neurologic status.
- Monitor the serum sodium level.
- Monitor urine specific gravity.
- Monitor fluid intake and output and daily weight measurements.

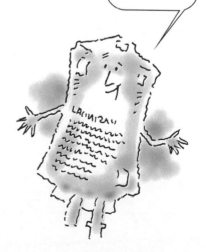

Use a salt-free I.V. solution.

Hyponatremia

Key facts

- Hyponatremia is characterized by a serum sodium level less than 135 mEq/L (SI, 135 mmol/L).
- In hyponatremia, body fluids are diluted and cells swell from decreased extracellular fluid osmolality.
- Severe hyponatremia (sodium level less than 110 mEq/L [SI, 110 mmol/L]) can lead to seizures, coma, and permanent neurologic damage.
- Hyponatremia can be triggered by sodium loss, water gain (dilutional hyponatremia), or inadequate sodium intake (depletional hyponatremia).
- Hyponatremia can be hypovolemic (with decreased extracellular fluid volume), hypervolemic (with increased extracellular fluid volume), or isovolumic (with extracellular fluid volume equal to intracellular fluid volume).

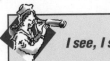

I see, I see

What happens in hyponatremia

Sodium loss or water gain increases or sodium intake decreases.

Fluid moves by osmosis from the extracellular space
(which has more water and less sodium)
into the more concentrated intracellular space.

Cells contain more fluid and blood vessels contain less.
Cerebral edema and hypovolemia can occur.

What causes it

- Hypovolemic hyponatremia
  - Osmotic diuresis
  - Salt-losing nephritis
  - Adrenal insufficiency
  - Diuretic use
  - Vomiting
  - Diarrhea
  - Fistulas
  - Gastric suctioning
  - Excessive diaphoresis
  - Cystic fibrosis
  - Burns
  - Wound drainage
- Hypervolemic hyponatremia
  - Heart or liver failure
  - Nephrotic syndrome
  - Excessive use of hypotonic fluids
  - Hyperaldosteronism
- Isovolumic hyponatremia
  - Glucocorticoid deficiency
  - Hypothyroidism
  - Renal failure
  - Syndrome of inappropriate antidiuretic hormone (SIADH)

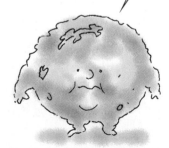

Do I look bloated to you?

Drugs that can cause hyponatremia

Anticonvulsants
- Carbamazepine

Antidiabetics
- Chlorpropamide
- Tolbutamide, rarely

Antineoplastics
- Cyclophosphamide
- Vincristine

Antipsychotics
- Fluphenazine
- Thioridazine
- Thiothixene

Diuretics
- Bumetanide
- Ethacrynic acid
- Furosemide

- Thiazides, such as chlorothiazide and hydrochlorothiazide

Sedatives
- Barbiturates, such as phenobarbital and secobarbital
- Morphine

What to look for
- Abdominal cramps
- Altered level of consciousness (LOC), such as lethargy and confusion
- Headache
- Muscle twitching, tremors, and weakness
- Nausea
- Seizures

Hyponatremia caused by hypovolemia
- Dry mucous membranes
- Orthostatic hypotension or low blood pressure
- Poor skin turgor
- Tachycardia
- Weak pulses

Hyponatremia caused by hypervolemia
- Edema
- Hypertension

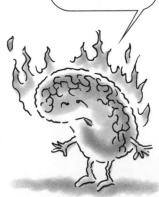

An altered LOC and headache are signs of hyponatremia.

- Rapid, bounding pulses
- Weight gain

What tests show
- Elevated hematocrit and plasma protein levels
- Serum osmolality less than 280 mOsm/kg (dilute blood)
- Serum sodium level less than 135 mEq/L (SI, 135 mmol/L)
- Urine specific gravity less than 1.010 (or increased urine specific gravity and urine sodium level in a patient with SIADH)

How it's treated

Mild hyponatremia with hypervolemia or isovolumia
- Restrict the patient's fluid intake.
- Provide oral sodium supplements.

Mild hyponatremia with hypovolemia
- Administer isotonic I.V. fluids, such as normal saline solution, to restore volume.
- Provide high-sodium foods.

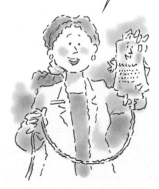

Give your patient isotonic I.V. fluids to treat mild hyponatremia with hypovolemia.

Severe hyponatremia

- Infuse a hypertonic solution, such as 3% or 5% saline solution, giving it slowly and in small volumes to prevent fluid overload.
- Watch for signs and symptoms of circulatory overload or worsening neurologic status.
- Hypervolemic patients shouldn't receive hypertonic sodium chloride solutions, except in rare instances of severe symptomatic hyponatremia.
- Monitor the serum sodium level to evaluate the patient's response to therapy.
- Monitor the patient's fluid intake and output and daily weight measurements.

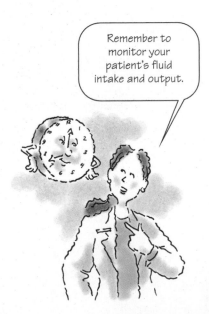

Remember to monitor your patient's fluid intake and output.

Hyperkalemia

Key facts

- Hyperkalemia is characterized by a serum potassium level greater than 5 mEq/L (SI, 5 mmol/L).
- In hyperkalemia, the body has an excess of potassium relative to water.
- Hyperkalemia is the most dangerous electrolyte disorder. Even a slight increase in the potassium level can profoundly affect the neuromuscular and cardiovascular systems.

I see, I see

What happens in hyperkalemia

Potassium intake increases or potassium excretion decreases.

▼

Potassium shifts out of cells into extracellular fluid.

▼

Extracellular potassium level rises.

▼

Patient develops neuromuscular and cardiac signs and symptoms.

What causes it

- Increased potassium intake
  - Overconsumption of dietary potassium
  - Excessive use of salt substitutes or potassium supplements
  - High-volume blood transfusion
  - Use of certain drugs
- Decreased potassium excretion
  - Acute or chronic renal failure
  - Disorders that damage the kidneys
  - Addison's disease
  - Hypoaldosteronism
- Potassium release from cells
  - Burns
  - Severe infection
  - Trauma
  - Crush injury
  - Intravascular hemolysis
  - Metabolic acidosis
  - Insulin deficiency

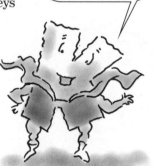

Too much potassium can lead to hyperkalemia.

Drugs that can cause hyperkalemia

- Angiotensin-converting enzyme inhibitors
- Antibiotics
- Beta-adrenergic blockers
- Chemotherapeutic drugs
- Nonsteroidal anti-inflammatory drugs
- Potassium, in excessive amounts
- Spironolactone

What to look for

- Abdominal cramps
- Decreased heart rate
- Diarrhea
- Hypotension
- Irregular pulse rate
- Irritability
- Muscle weakness, especially in the legs
- Nausea
- Paresthesia

What tests show

- Decreased arterial pH, indicating acidosis
- Electrocardiogram (ECG) changes, especially tall, tented T waves and, possibly, flattened P waves, prolonged PR intervals, widened QRS complexes, and depressed ST segments
- Serum potassium level greater than 5 mEq/L (SI, 5 mmol/L)

How it's treated

- Restrict the patient's potassium intake.
- Stop or readjust drugs that may be contributing to hyperkalemia.
- Treat mild cases with a loop diuretic such as furosemide.
- For a patient with renal failure, diuretics may not be effective. If so, plan to use hemodialysis or a similar therapy to lower the potassium level.
- Administer sodium polystyrene sulfonate by mouth, via nasogastric (NG) tube, or as a retention enema. Give this drug with sorbitol or another osmotic substance to promote its excretion.

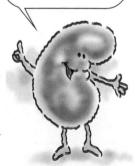

Diuretics may not be effective in treating a patient with renal failure who has developed hyperkalemia.

- Closely monitor the patient's cardiac status, including ECG tracings.
- Administer 10% calcium gluconate to counteract the myocardial effects of hyperkalemia.
- Administer regular insulin and hypertonic dextrose by I.V. to move potassium into the cells. During therapy, monitor for hypoglycemia.
- Administer sodium bicarbonate to a patient with acidosis to shift potassium into the cells.
- Closely monitor the patient's fluid intake and output.
- If the patient doesn't respond to treatment, prepare him for dialysis.

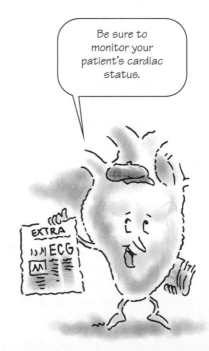

Hypokalemia

Key facts

- Hypokalemia is characterized by a serum potassium level less than 3.5 mEq/L (SI, 3.5 mmol/L).
- In hypokalemia, potassium deficiency occurs because the body can't effectively conserve potassium.

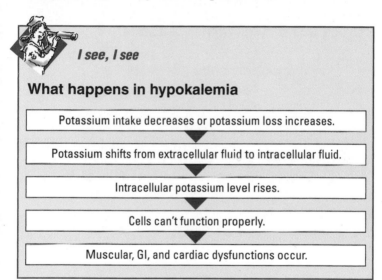

I see, I see

What happens in hypokalemia

Potassium intake decreases or potassium loss increases.

Potassium shifts from extracellular fluid to intracellular fluid.

Intracellular potassium level rises.

Cells can't function properly.

Muscular, GI, and cardiac dysfunctions occur.

What causes it

- Inadequate potassium intake
  - Low consumption of potassium-rich foods
  - Use of potassium-deficient I.V. fluids
- Excessive potassium output
  - Severe GI fluid loss (as with suction, lavage, prolonged vomiting, or diarrhea)
  - Severe diaphoresis

– Diuresis (as with recent kidney transplantation or a high urine glucose level)
– Use of certain drugs
– Renal tubular acidosis
– Magnesium depletion
– Cushing's syndrome
– Stress

Drugs that can cause hypokalemia

- Adrenergics, such as albuterol and epinephrine
- Antibiotics, such as amphotericin B, carbenicillin, and gentamicin
- Cisplatin
- Corticosteroids
- Diuretics, such as furosemide and thiazides
- Insulin
- Laxatives, with excessive use

What to look for

- Anorexia
- Constipation
- Hyporeflexia
- Muscle cramps and weakness
- Nausea and vomiting
- Orthostatic hypotension
- Paresthesia
- Polyuria
- Weak, irregular pulses

What tests show

- Elevated pH and bicarbonate levels
- ECG changes, such as flattened T waves, depressed ST segments, and characteristic U waves
- Serum potassium level less than 3.5 mEq/L (SI, 3.5 mmol/L)
- Slightly elevated serum glucose level

How it's treated

- Focus treatment on restoring potassium balance, removing the underlying cause, and preventing complications, such as arrhythmias, cardiac arrest, and respiratory arrest.
- Place the patient on a high-potassium diet.
- Provide oral potassium supplements as needed.
- To prevent gastric irritation from oral potassium supplements, administer them in at least 4 oz (118 ml) of fluid or with food.
- To prevent a quick load of potassium from entering the body, don't crush slow-release potassium tablets.
- If the patient can't tolerate oral potassium supplements or has severe hypokalemia, administer I.V. potassium, using an infusion pump to control the flow rate.
- Never give potassium by I.V. push or bolus because such rapid administration could be fatal.
- When selecting a vein for I.V. therapy, remember that potassium preparations can irritate peripheral veins and cause discomfort. When possible, choose a more

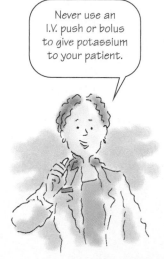

Never use an I.V. push or bolus to give potassium to your patient.

proximal site, such as an antecubital vein rather than a vein in the hand.

- Consider switching the patient to a potassium-sparing diuretic if indicated.
- Monitor the patient's vital signs, particularly noting orthostatic hypotension.
- Monitor the patient's heart rate and rhythm if his potassium level is less than 3 mEq/L (SI, 3 mmol/L) or if the I.V. potassium infusion exceeds 5 mEq/hour (SI, 5 mmol/h).
- Assess the patient's respiratory status because hypokalemia can weaken or paralyze respiratory muscles. Keep a manual resuscitation bag at the bedside.

Hypermagnesemia

Key facts

- Hypermagnesemia is characterized by a serum magnesium level greater than 2.1 mg/dl (SI, 1.05 mmol/L).

I see, I see

What happens in hypermagnesemia

Magnesium excretion decreases or magnesium intake increases.

▼

High magnesium level suppresses acetylcholine release at myoneural junctions.

▼

Reduced acetylcholine blocks neuromuscular transmission and reduces cell excitability.

▼

The neuromuscular and central nervous systems become depressed.

▼

LOC decreases and respiratory distress occurs.

▼

Arrhythmias and other cardiac complications may develop.

What causes it

- Impaired magnesium excretion
  - Renal dysfunction
  - Advanced age
  - Renal failure
  - Addison's disease
  - Adrenocortical insufficiency

– Diabetic ketoacidosis (DKA)
- Excessive magnesium intake
    – Use of certain drugs
    – Use of magnesium-rich dialysate for hemodialysis
    – Use of magnesium-rich solutions for total parenteral nutrition (TPN)
    – Treatment with continuous infusion of magnesium sulfate

---

Drugs that can cause hypermagnesemia

- Antacids such as magnesium-aluminum combination drugs
- Laxatives that contain magnesium (magnesium citrate)
- Magnesium supplements, such as magnesium oxide and magnesium sulfate

---

What to look for

- Bradycardia, possibly leading to heart block and cardiac arrest
- Decreased LOC, progressing from drowsiness and lethargy to coma
- Decreased muscle and nerve activity
- Flushed skin and feelings of warmth
- Hypoactive deep tendon reflexes (DTRs)
- Hypotension
- Generalized weakness
- Nausea and vomiting
- Respirations that are slow, shallow, and depressed
- Respiratory arrest

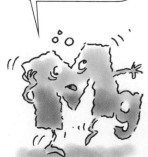

The use of magnesium-rich solutions can cause hypermagnesemia.

Through the ages

Pediatric magnesium levels

Magnesium levels in pediatric patients differ from those in adults. In newborns, the normal magnesium level ranges from 1.5 to 2.2 mg/dl (SI, 0.62 to 0.91 mmol/L); in children, from 1.7 to 2.1 mg/dl (SI, 0.70 to 0.86 mmol/L).

What tests show

- ECG changes, such as prolonged PR intervals, widened QRS complexes, and tall T waves
- Serum magnesium level greater than 2.6 mEq/L (SI, 1.07 mmol/L)

How it's treated

- If the patient has normal renal function, administer oral or I.V. fluids to rid the body of excessive magnesium.
- If fluid administration isn't effective, give a loop diuretic, such as furosemide, to promote magnesium excretion.
- In an emergency, administer calcium gluconate (a magnesium antagonist).
- Provide mechanical ventilation if hypermagnesemia compromises respiratory function.

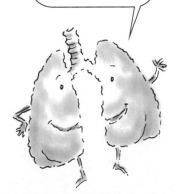

If your patient suffers from hypermagnesemia, take a close look at his respiratory functioning.

- For a patient with severe renal dysfunction, prepare for hemodialysis with a magnesium-free dialysate solution.
- Assess the patient's DTRs and muscle strength. Also assess his skin for flushing and diaphoresis.
- Closely monitor the patient's respiratory status.
- Monitor for fluid overload if the patient receives large volumes of fluid.
- Avoid the use of drugs that contain magnesium, and restrict the patient's dietary intake of magnesium.
- Closely monitor the patient receiving magnesium sulfate. Also monitor the neonate of a mother who received magnesium sulfate for hypertension or preterm labor.

Hypomagnesemia

Key facts

- Hypomagnesemia is characterized by a serum magnesium level less than 1.3 mg/dl (SI, 0.65 mmol/L).
- This relatively common condition can lead to respiratory muscle paralysis, complete heart block, and coma.

I see, I see

What happens in hypomagnesemia

Magnesium intake or absorption decreases or magnesium loss increases.

Magnesium moves out of cells to compensate for low extracellular magnesium level.

Cells become starved for magnesium.

Skeletal muscles weaken, and nerves and muscles become hyperirritable.

What causes it

- Inadequate magnesium intake
  - Chronic alcoholism
  - Prolonged I.V. fluid therapy
  - Use of TPN or enteral feeding formulas without sufficient magnesium
- Inadequate GI absorption of magnesium
  - Malabsorption syndrome
  - Steatorrhea
  - Ulcerative colitis
  - Crohn's disease
  - Bowel resection or similar GI surgery
  - Cancer
  - Pancreatic insufficiency
  - Excess calcium or phosphorus in the GI tract
- Excessive GI loss of magnesium
  - Prolonged diarrhea
  - Fistula drainage
  - Laxative abuse
  - NG tube suctioning
  - Acute pancreatitis
- Excessive urinary loss of magnesium
  - Primary aldosteronism
  - Hyperparathyroidism or hypoparathyroidism
  - DKA
  - Use of certain drugs
  - Renal disorders, such as glomerulonephritis, pyelonephritis, and renal tubular acidosis

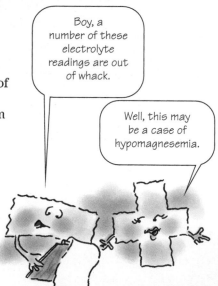

Drugs that can cause hypomagnesemia

- Aminoglycoside antibiotics, such as amikacin, gentamicin, streptomycin, and tobramycin
- Amphotericin B
- Cisplatin
- Cyclosporine
- Insulin
- Laxatives
- Loop diuretics, such as bumetanide, furosemide, and torsemide
- Pentamidine isethionate
- Thiazide diuretics, such as chlorothiazide and hydrochlorothiazide

What to look for

- Altered LOC and confusion, hallucinations, or seizures
- Anorexia and dysphagia
- Arrhythmias, such as atrial fibrillation, heart block, paroxysmal atrial tachycardia, premature ventricular contractions, supraventricular tachycardia, torsades de pointes, ventricular fibrillation, and ventricular tachycardia
- Chvostek's sign and Trousseau's sign
- Hyperactive DTRs
- Hypertension
- Leg and foot cramps
- Muscle weakness, twitching, tremors, or tetany
- Nausea and vomiting
- Respiratory difficulties

What tests show

- ECG changes, such as prolonged PR intervals, widened QRS complexes, prolonged QT intervals, depressed ST segments, broad flattened T waves, and prominent U waves
- Elevated serum digoxin level in a patient receiving the drug
- Serum magnesium level less than 1.3 mg/dl (SI, 0.65 mmol/L), possibly with a below normal serum albumin level

- Other electrolyte abnormalities, such as a below normal serum potassium or calcium level

How it's treated

- Manage a mild deficiency with increased intake of magnesium-rich foods or with oral supplements. Continue oral magnesium replacement for several days after the serum magnesium level returns to normal.
- Treat a severe deficiency with I.V. or deep I.M. injections of magnesium sulfate.
- Before administering magnesium, assess the patient's renal function. If renal function is impaired (urine output less than 10 ml in 4 hours), monitor the magnesium level closely because the kidneys excrete this electrolyte.
- Monitor the patient's neuromuscular status to detect hyperactive DTRs, tremors, and tetany.
- Check for Chvostek's and Trousseau's signs.
- Assess for dysphagia before giving the patient food.
- Monitor the patient's respiratory status, which can be compromised by hypomagnesemia-induced laryngeal stridor and breathing difficulty.
- Regularly assess the patient's urine output.
- If the patient receives digoxin, monitor for signs and symptoms of digoxin toxicity because hypomagnesemia can increase the risk of this adverse reaction.
- Monitor all electrolyte levels because hypocalcemia and hypokalemia can cause hypomagnesemia, especially if the patient receives a diuretic.
- Institute seizure precautions as needed.

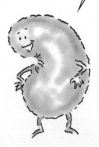

Don't forget to assess your patient's renal function.

Hypercalcemia

Key facts

- Hypercalcemia is characterized by a total serum calcium level greater than 10.2 mg/dl (SI, 2.54 mmol/L) and an ionized serum calcium level greater than 5.28 mg/dl (SI, 1.25 mmol/L).
- In hypercalcemia, the rate of calcium entry into extracellular fluid exceeds the rate of calcium excretion by the kidneys.

I see, I see

What happens in hypercalcemia

Calcium resorption from bone increases.

▼

Calcium enters extracellular fluid at an increased rate.

Calcium movement into extracellular fluid exceeds the rate of calcium excretion by the kidneys.

Excess calcium enters cells.

Excess intracellular calcium decreases cell membrane excitability.

Reduced membrane excitability affects skeletal and cardiac muscles and the nervous system.

▼

Patient may display fatigue, confusion, and decreased level of consciousness.

What causes it

- Increased calcium resorption from bone
  - Hyperparathyroidism
  - Cancer
- Use of certain drugs
- Increased calcium absorption or decreased calcium excretion
  - Hyperthyroidism
  - Multiple fractures
  - Prolonged immobilization
  - Hypophosphatemia
  - Acidosis

Drugs that can cause hypercalcemia

- Antacids that contain calcium
- Calcium preparations (oral or I.V.)
- Lithium
- Thiazide diuretics, such as chlorothiazide and hydrochlorothiazide
- Vitamin A
- Vitamin D

What to look for

- Abdominal pain and constipation
- Anorexia
- Behavioral changes, including confusion
- Bone pain
- Decreased LOC, which may progress from lethargy to coma
- Extreme thirst and polyuria
- Hypertension
- Hypoactive DTRs
- Muscle weakness
- Nausea and vomiting

Through the ages

Pediatric calcium levels

Pediatric patients normally have higher serum calcium levels than adults. In fact, their serum calcium levels can rise as high as 11.2 mg/dl (SI, 2.79 mmol/L) during periods of increased bone growth. Geriatric patients normally have a narrower range of normal calcium levels than younger adults do. For older men, the range is 2.3 to 3.7 mg/dl (SI, 0.57 to 0.92 mmol/L); for older women, it's 2.8 to 4.1 mg/dl (SI, 0.25 to 1.02 mmol/L).

What tests show

- ECG changes, such as shortened QT intervals and shortened ST segments
- Elevated serum digoxin level in a patient receiving the drug
- Ionized calcium level greater than 5.28 mg/dl (SI, 1.25 mmol/L)
- Total serum calcium level greater than 10.2 mg/dl (SI, 2.54 mmol/L)
- X-rays revealing pathologic fractures

How it's treated

- Limit the patient's dietary calcium intake and discontinue drugs or infusions that contain calcium.
- Hydrate the patient with normal saline solution to promote diuresis and calcium excretion.

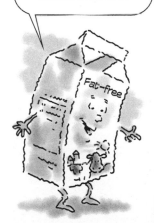

If your patient has hypercalcemia, limit calcium in his diet.

Fat-free

- Administer a loop diuretic, such as furosemide, to help promote calcium excretion.
- Don't give a thiazide diuretic to a patient with hypercalcemia because it can inhibit calcium excretion.
- For a patient with life-threatening hypercalcemia, prepare for dialysis.
- Administer a corticosteroid as prescribed to block bone resorption and decrease GI absorption of calcium.
- Give etidronate disodium as prescribed to inhibit the action of osteoclasts in the bone. For hypercalcemia caused by cancer, give plicamycin.
- Assess the patient for arrhythmias.
- Assess for signs and symptoms of renal calculi; strain the patient's urine if needed.
- Assess for signs and symptoms of digoxin toxicity if the patient also receives digoxin.

Hypocalcemia

Key facts

- Hypocalcemia is characterized by a total serum calcium level less than 8.2 mg/dl (SI, 2.05 mmol/L) and an ionized serum calcium level less than 4.6 mg/dl (SI, 1.1 mmol/L).

I see, I see

What happens in hypocalcemia

Calcium or vitamin D intake or absorption decreases or calcium excretion increases.

Parathyroid glands release parathyroid hormone (PTH).

PTH draws calcium from bone and promotes renal reabsorption and intestinal absorption of calcium.

Lack of calcium outstrips PTH's ability to compensate.

Calcium is no longer available to maintain cell structure and function.

Patient develops neuromuscular and cardiac symptoms and decreased level of consciousness.

What causes it

- Inadequate calcium intake
  - Chronic alcoholism
  - Insufficient exposure to sunlight
  - Possibly breast-feeding
- Calcium malabsorption
  - Severe diarrhea
  - Laxative abuse
  - Malabsorption syndrome
  - Insufficient vitamin D
  - High phosphorus level in the intestines
  - Reduced gastric acidity
- Excess calcium loss
  - Pancreatic insufficiency
  - Acute pancreatitis
  - Thyroid or parathyroid surgery
  - Hypoparathyroidism or other parathyroid gland disorders
  - Use of certain drugs
- Other causes
  - Severe burns and infections

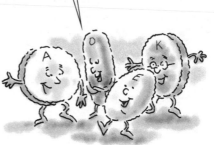

If you don't get enough of me, you risk hypocalcemia.

Drugs that can cause hypocalcemia

- Anticonvulsants, especially phenytoin and phenobarbital
- Calcitonin
- Drugs that lower the serum magnesium level, such as cisplatin and gentamicin
- Edetate disodium
- Loop diuretics, such as ethacrynic acid and furosemide
- Plicamycin
- Phosphates (oral, I.V., or rectal)

Through the ages

Geriatric calcium levels

Factors that contribute to hypocalcemia in geriatric patients include inadequate dietary intake of calcium, poor calcium absorption, and reduced activity or inactivity.

– Hypoalbuminemia
– Hyperphosphatemia
– Alkalosis
– Massive blood transfusion

What to look for
• Anxiety, confusion, and irritability
• Arrhythmias and decreased cardiac output
• Brittle nails or dry skin and hair
• Diarrhea
• Diminished response to digoxin
• Hyperactive DTRs
• Paresthesia of toes, fingers, or face, especially around the mouth
• Spasms of laryngeal and abdominal muscles
• Tetany, tremors, twitching, and muscle cramps
• Trousseau's sign or Chvostek's sign

What tests show
• ECG changes, such as lengthened QT intervals and prolonged ST segments
• Ionized calcium level less than 4.6 mg/dl (SI, 1.1 mmol/L)
• Total serum calcium level less than 8.2 mg/dl (SI, 2.05 mmol/L)

Through the ages

Breast-feeding and hypocalcemia

A breast-fed infant can develop low calcium and vitamin D levels if the mother's intake of these nutrients is inadequate.

How it's treated

- For a patient with acute hypocalcemia, immediately administer I.V. calcium gluconate or calcium chloride.
- Frequently assess the I.V. site and administer I.V. calcium with an infusion pump because infiltration can cause tissue necrosis and sloughing. Never administer I.V. calcium rapidly because it may cause syncope, hypotension, and arrhythmias.
- Give magnesium with calcium because hypocalcemia doesn't respond to calcium therapy alone.
- For a patient with chronic hypocalcemia, begin vitamin D supplementation to promote calcium absorption.
- Provide a diet that's rich in calcium, vitamin D, and protein.
- Administer a phosphate binder, such as an aluminum hydroxide antacid, to lower an elevated phosphorus level, if needed.

Be sure not to administer I.V. calcium to your patient too quickly. Remember, slow and steady treats hypocalcemia.

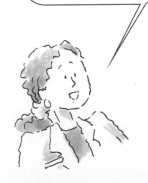

Checking for Trousseau's and Chvostek's signs

Testing for Trousseau's and Chvostek's signs can aid in the diagnosis of tetany and hypocalcemia.

Trousseau's sign

To check for Trousseau's sign, apply a blood pressure cuff to the patient's upper arm and inflate it to a pressure 20 mm Hg above the systolic pressure. Trousseau's sign may appear after 1 to 4 minutes. The patient will experience an adducted thumb, flexed wrist and metacarpophalangeal joints, and extended interphalangeal joints (with fingers together)—carpopedal spasm—indicating tetany, a major sign of hypocalcemia.

Chvostek's sign

You can induce Chvostek's sign by tapping the patient's facial nerve adjacent to the ear. A brief contraction of the upper lip, nose, or side of the face indicates Chvostek's sign and tetany.

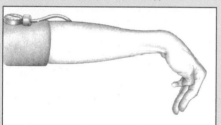
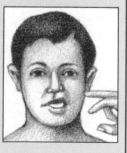

- Keep a tracheotomy tray and handheld resuscitation bag nearby in case the patient develops laryngospasm.
- Place the patient on a cardiac monitor to detect changes in heart rate and rhythm, especially if he's receiving digoxin.
- Assess for Chvostek's sign and Trousseau's sign.
- Institute seizure precautions if indicated.

Hyperphosphatemia

Key facts

- Hyperphosphatemia is characterized by a serum phosphorus level greater than 4.5 mg/dl (SI, 1.45 mmol/L).

I see, I see

What happens in hyperphosphatemia

Intake of phosphorus or vitamin D is excessive.	Renal insult or failure reduces glomerular filtration rate to below 30 ml/minute.

Kidneys can't filter excess phosphorus adequately.

Phosphorus shifts from intracelluar to extracellular fluid.

Serum phosphorus level increases.

Phosphorus binds with calcium, forming insoluble compound.

Insoluble compound is deposited in lungs, heart, kidneys, eyes, skin, and other soft tissues.

What causes it

- Impaired phosphorus excretion
  - Hypoparathyroidism
  - Any disorder that causes the glomerular filtration rate to fall below 30 ml/minute
- Phosphorus shifting to extracellular fluid
  - Acid-base imbalances
  - Chemotherapy
  - Muscle necrosis
  - Rhabdomyolysis
- Increased phosphorus intake
  - Overuse of phosphorus supplements
  - Overuse of phosphorus-containing laxatives or enemas
  - Use of certain drugs

Drugs that can cause hyperphosphatemia

- Enemas containing phosphorus
- Laxatives containing phosphorus or phosphate
- Oral phosphorus supplements
- Parenteral phosphorus supplements, such as sodium phosphate and potassium phosphate
- Vitamin D supplements

What to look for

- Anorexia, nausea, and vomiting
- Arrhythmias and irregular heart rate
- Chvostek's sign or Trousseau's sign
- Conjunctivitis or vision impairment
- Impaired mental status and seizures
- Hyperreflexia
- Muscle weakness, cramps, and spasms
- Papular eruptions and dry, itchy skin

Through the ages

Cow's milk and hyperphosphatemia

Infants who are fed cow's milk are predisposed to hyperphosphatemia because cow's milk contains more phosphorus than breast milk.

- Paresthesia, especially in the fingertips and around the mouth
- Tetany

What tests show

- ECG changes, such as prolonged QT intervals and ST segments
- Increased blood urea nitrogen and creatinine levels, which reflect worsening renal function
- Serum calcium level less than 8.2 mg/dl (SI, 2.05 mmol/L)
- Serum phosphorus level less than 4.5 mg/dl (SI, 1.45 mmol/L)
- Phosphorus and calcium have an inverse relationship, meaning that hyperphosphatemia may lead to hypocalcemia, which can be life-threatening
- X-rays revealing skeletal changes caused by osteodystrophy in chronic hyperphosphatemia

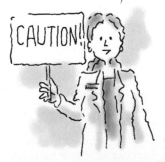

Hyperphosphatemia may lead to hypocalcemia.

CAUTION!

How it's treated

- Limit the patient's phosphorus intake from dietary sources or drugs.
- Give an aluminum, magnesium, or calcium gel or phosphorus-binding antacid to decrease GI absorption of phosphorus.
- For a patient with renal insufficiency, avoid the use of magnesium antacids because of the increased risk of hypermagnesemia.
- Treat the underlying cause of hyperphosphatemia, such as respiratory acidosis or DKA, which can lower the serum phosphorus level.
- For a patient with severe hyperphosphatemia and normal renal function, administer I.V. saline solution to promote renal excretion of phosphorus.
- If hyperphosphatemia is related to renal failure, prepare the patient for dialysis.
- Monitor the patient for signs and symptoms of calcium phosphate calcification.
- Monitor for signs and symptoms of hypocalcemia.

Signs of calcification

Calcification usually results from chronic elevation of the serum phosphorus level. It can produce these signs:
- arrhythmias
- conjunctivitis
- corneal haziness and impaired vision
- decreased urine output
- irregular heart rate or palpitations
- papular eruptions.

Hypophosphatemia

Key facts

- Hypophosphatemia is characterized by a serum phosphorus level less than 2.7 mg/dl (SI, 0.87 mmol/L).
- Generally, hypophosphatemia indicates a phosphorus deficiency. However, it can occur under circumstances when total body phosphorus stores are normal.
- Severe hypophosphatemia occurs when the serum phosphorus level is less than 1 mg/dl (SI, 0.3 mmol/L) and can lead to organ failure.

I see, I see

What happens in hypophosphatemia

Intestinal absorption decreases.	Renal elimination increases.	Phosphorus moves from extracellular fluid into the cells.

▼ ▼ ▼

Phosphorus level decreases.

▼

Cellular energy stores decrease because of adenosine triphosphate (ATP) depletion.

▼

Patient develops musculoskeletal, neurologic, cardiac, and hematologic effects.

What causes it

- Phosphorus shifting to intracellular fluid
  - Respiratory alkalosis
  - Hyperglycemia
  - Insulin therapy
  - Malnourishment
  - Hypothermia
- Decreased phosphorus absorption
  - Malabsorption syndromes
  - Starvation
  - Prolonged or excessive use of phosphorus-binding antacids
  - Inadequate vitamin D intake or synthesis
  - Diarrhea
  - Laxative abuse
- Increased renal loss of phosphorus
  - Diuretic use
  - DKA
  - Alcohol abuse
  - Hyperparathyroidism
  - Hypocalcemia
  - Extensive burns

Drugs that can cause hypophosphatemia

- Diuretics, such as acetazolamide, loop diuretics (bumetanide and furosemide), and thiazide diuretics (chlorothiazide and hydrochloro-thiazide)
- Antacids, such as aluminum carbonate, aluminum hydroxide, calcium carbonate, and magnesium oxide
- Insulin
- Laxatives
- Phosphorus-binding drugs, such as sevelamer and calcium acetate

Through the ages

Geriatric laxative use

A geriatric patient's drugs can alter electrolyte levels by affecting phosphorus absorption. Be sure to ask if the patient uses over-the-counter drugs, such as antacids or laxatives.

What to look for

- Anorexia
- Bruising and bleeding, particularly mild GI bleeding
- Chest pain
- Hypotension and low cardiac output
- Irritability, apprehension, and confusion
- Muscle weakness, myalgia, and malaise
- Osteomalacia and bone pain
- Paresthesia
- Respiratory failure
- Seizures and coma

What tests show

- Elevated creatine kinase level, if rhabdomyolysis is present
- Serum phosphorus level less than 2.7 mg/dl (SI, 0.87 mmol/L)
- X-rays revealing skeletal changes caused by osteomalacia or bone fractures

How it's treated

- If hypophosphatemia is mild, encourage the patient to eat a high-phosphorus diet.
- If the patient has moderate hypophosphatemia or can't consume phosphorus-rich foods, provide oral supplements.

- If hypophosphatemia is severe, replace the deficient electrolyte with I.V. potassium phosphate or sodium phosphate.
- Administer potassium phosphate slowly (no faster than 10 mEq/hour [SI, 10 mmol/h]). Adverse effects of too-rapid I.V. replacement for hypophosphatemia include hyperphosphatemia and hypocalcemia.
- Assess the patient's medication history.
- Monitor for "refeeding syndrome" when a patient starts TPN therapy. This syndrome, which causes phosphorus to shift into cells, usually occurs 3 or more days after TPN begins.
- Closely monitor the results of arterial blood gas analysis and pulse oximetry to detect respiratory changes.
- Closely monitor the patient's cardiac and neurologic status.
- Institute seizure precautions if needed.

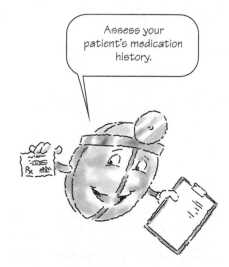

Assess your patient's medication history.

Hyperchloremia

Key facts

- Hyperchloremia is characterized by a serum chloride level greater than 106 mEq/L (SI, 106 mmol/L).
- In hyperchloremia, excess chloride in extracellular fluid is linked to other electrolyte imbalances. Therefore, it rarely occurs alone.

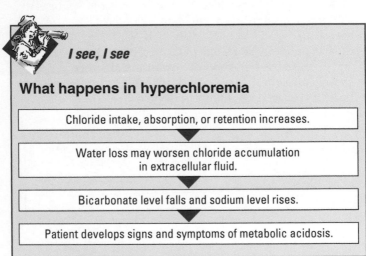

I see, I see

What happens in hyperchloremia

Chloride intake, absorption, or retention increases.

Water loss may worsen chloride accumulation in extracellular fluid.

Bicarbonate level falls and sodium level rises.

Patient develops signs and symptoms of metabolic acidosis.

What causes it

- Increased chloride intake or absorption
  - Overconsumption of sodium chloride
  - Water loss
  - Anastomoses of the ureter and intestines
- Acidosis
  - Dehydration
  - Renal tubular acidosis

  - Renal failure
  - Respiratory alkalosis
  - Salicylate toxicity
  - Hyperparathyroidism
  - Hyperaldosteronism
  - Hypernatremia
- Chloride retention by the kidneys
  - Use of certain drugs

Drugs that can cause hyperchloremia

- Acetazolamide
- Ammonium chloride
- Phenylbutazone
- Salicylates, such as aspirin, with overdose
- Sodium polystyrene sulfonate
- Triamterene

What to look for

- Arrhythmias and decreased cardiac output
- Decreased LOC, possibly progressing to coma
- Dyspnea
- Fluid retention and edema
- Kussmaul's respirations
- Lethargy
- Other signs and symptoms of metabolic acidosis
- Tachycardia and hypertension
- Tachypnea
- Weakness

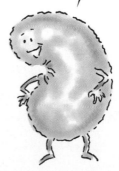

If I retain chloride, it can lead to hyperchloremia.

Through the ages

Geriatric chloride levels

In patients between ages 60 and 90, the normal serum chloride level ranges from 98 to 107 mEq/L (SI, 98 to 107 mmol/L); in patients age 90 and older, from 98 to 111 mEq/L (SI, 98 to 111 mmol/L).

What tests show

- Serum chloride level greater than 106 mEq/L (SI, 106 mmol/L)
- Serum pH less than 7.35 (SI, 7.35), serum bicarbonate level less than 22 mEq/L (SI, 22 mmol/L), and normal anion gap (8 to 14 mEq/L [SI, 8 to 14 mmol/L]), suggesting metabolic acidosis
- Serum sodium level greater than 145 mEq/L (SI, 145 mmol/L)

How it's treated

- Focus on restoring the patient's fluid, electrolyte, and acid-base balance.
- Restrict the patient's sodium and chloride intake.
- Administer a diuretic to promote chloride elimination, if the patient isn't dehydrated.
- For a dehydrated patient, administer fluids to dilute the blood and force renal excretion of chloride.
- In a patient with adequate liver function, correct acidosis by infusing lactated Ringer's solution as prescribed.
- If hyperchloremia is severe, administer I.V. sodium bicarbonate to raise the serum bicarbonate level.
- Closely monitor the patient's cardiac rhythm to detect changes.
- If the patient is receiving I.V. bicarbonate, monitor for signs and symptoms of metabolic alkalosis, which may result from overcorrection.

Hypochloremia

Key facts

- Hypochloremia is characterized by a serum chloride level less than 96 mEq/L (SI, 96 mmol/L).
- In hypochloremia, a chloride deficiency exists in extracellular fluid.
- A decrease in the serum chloride level can affect the levels of sodium, potassium, calcium, and other electrolytes.

I see, I see

What happens in hypochloremia

Chloride intake or absorption decreases or chloride loss increases.

▼

Kidneys retain sodium and bicarbonate ions.

▼

Bicarbonate ions accumulate in extracellular fluid.

▼

Excess bicarbonate raises the pH.

▼

Hypochloremic metabolic alkalosis can occur.

▼

Patient displays arrhythmias, seizures, coma, and respiratory arrest.

What causes it
- Decreased chloride intake
  - Use of chloride-deficient formula in infants
  - Salt-restricted diet
  - Therapy with I.V. fluids that lack chloride
- Increased chloride loss
  - Prolonged vomiting
  - Diarrhea
  - Severe diaphoresis
  - Gastric surgery
  - NG tube suctioning
  - Other GI tube drainage
  - Cystic fibrosis
  - Use of certain drugs
- Other causes
  - Sodium deficiency
  - Potassium deficiency
  - Metabolic alkalosis
  - Conditions that affect acid-base or electrolyte balance, such as DKA, Addison's disease, and heart failure

Drugs that can cause hypochloremia
- Loop diuretics such as furosemide
- Osmotic diuretics such as mannitol
- Thiazide diuretics such as hydrochlorothiazide

What to look for
- Agitation and irritability
- Arrhythmias
- Hyperactive DTRs
- Muscle cramps and weakness
- Muscle hypertonicity
- Seizures or coma

- Slow, shallow respirations or respiratory arrest
- Other signs and symptoms of metabolic alkalosis
- Tetany
- Twitching

What tests show

- Serum chloride level less than 96 mEq/L (96 mmol/L)
- Serum pH greater than 7.45 (SI, 7.45) and serum bicarbonate level greater than 26 mEq/L (SI, 26 mmol/L), suggesting metabolic alkalosis
- Serum sodium level less than 135 mEq/L (SI 135 mmol/L), indicating hyponatremia

How it's treated

- Replace chloride by administering I.V. fluids, such as normal saline solution, or drugs and encouraging increased dietary intake of chloride.
- Treat accompanying metabolic alkalosis or electrolyte imbalances as indicated.
- Treat the underlying cause of renal or GI loss of chloride, for example, by withholding a diuretic or giving an antiemetic.
- Monitor the patient's LOC, muscle strength, and movement.
- Observe for worsening respiratory function. Keep emergency equipment nearby.

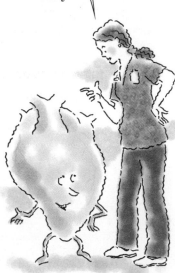

I need to monitor your rhythm. And-a-one-and-a-two...

- Monitor the patient's cardiac rhythm.
- If administering ammonium chloride to correct metabolic acidosis, assess the patient for pain at the infusion site and adjust the rate if needed.
- Don't give ammonium chloride to a patient with severe hepatic disease because the drug is metabolized by the liver.
- Use normal saline solution—not tap water—to flush the patient's NG tube.

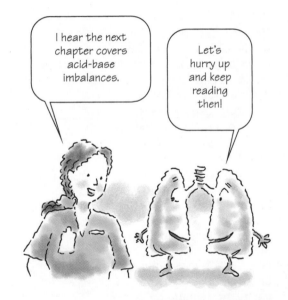

Acid-base imbalances

4

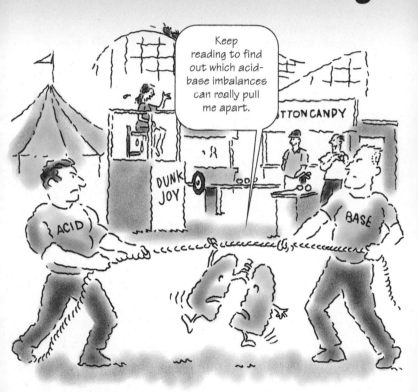

Respiratory acidosis

Key facts

- A compromise in any essential part of breathing—ventilation, perfusion, or diffusion—may lead to respiratory acidosis.
- In respiratory acidosis, the pulmonary system can't rid the body of enough carbon dioxide (CO_2) to maintain a healthy pH (hydrogen ion [H^+]) balance.
- Respiratory acidosis may be acute, in which pH falls abnormally low (less than 7.35 [SI, 7.35]).
- Respiratory acidosis may be chronic, in which pH stays within normal limits (7.34 to 7.45 [SI, 7.34 to 7.45]) because the kidneys have time to compensate for the imbalance.

Respiratory acidosis can be either acute or chronic.

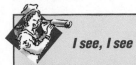

I see, I see

What happens in respiratory acidosis

This series of illustrations shows how respiratory acidosis develops at the cellular level.

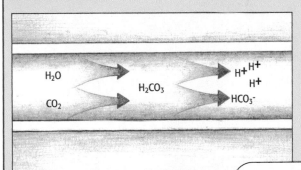

Step 1

When pulmonary ventilation decreases, retained CO_2 combines with water to form carbonic acid (H_2CO_3) in larger than normal amounts. The H_2CO_3 dissociates to release free hydrogen ions (H^+) and bicarbonate (HCO_3^-) ions. The excess H_2CO_3 causes a drop in pH. *Look for a $Paco_2$ level greater than 45 mm Hg (SI, 5.3 kPa) and a pH level less than 7.35 (SI, 7.35).*

> Follow the 6 steps to understand respiratory acidosis.

(continued)

What happens in respiratory acidosis *(continued)*

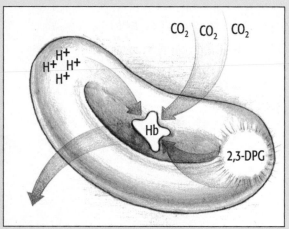

Step 2

As the pH level falls, 2,3-diphosphoglycerate (2,3-DPG) increases in the red blood cells (RBCs) and causes a change in hemoglobin (Hb) that makes the Hb release O_2. The altered Hb, now strongly alkaline, picks up H^+ and CO_2, thus eliminating some of the free H^+ and excess CO_2. *Look for decreased arterial O_2.*

Look for a decrease in arterial O_2.

What happens in respiratory acidosis *(continued)*

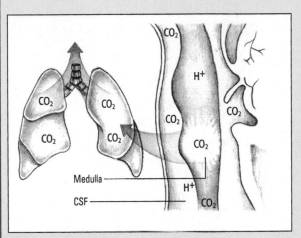

Step 3

Whenever $Paco_2$ increases, CO_2 builds up in all tissues and fluids, including cerebrospinal fluid (CSF) and the respiratory center in the medulla. The CO_2 reacts with H_2O to form H_2CO_3, which then breaks into free H^+ and HCO_3^- ions. The increased amount of CO_2 and free H^+ stimulate the respiratory center to increase the respiratory rate. An increased respiratory rate expels more CO_2 and helps to reduce the CO_2 level in the blood and other tissues. *Look for rapid, shallow respirations and a decreasing $Paco_2$.*

You're halfway there. Keep going!

(continued)

What happens in respiratory acidosis *(continued)*

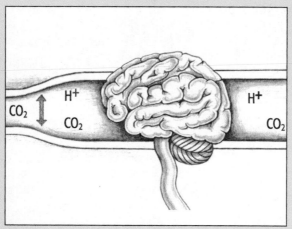

Step 4
Eventually, CO_2 and H^+ cause cerebral blood vessels to dilate, which increases blood flow to the brain. That increased flow can cause cerebral edema and depress CNS activity. *Look for headache, confusion, lethargy, nausea, or vomiting.*

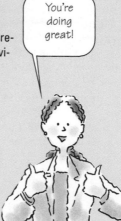

You're doing great!

What happens in respiratory acidosis (continued)

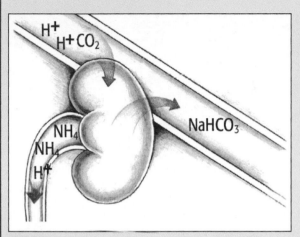

Step 5

As respiratory mechanisms fail, the increasing $Paco_2$ stimulates the kidneys to conserve HCO_3^- ions and Na^+ and to excrete H^+, partially in the form of ammonium (NH_4). The additional HCO_3^- and Na combine to form extra $NaHCO_3$, which is then able to buffer more free H^+. *Look for increased acid content in the urine, increasing serum pH and HCO_3^- levels, and shallow, depressed respirations.*

Only one more step to go!

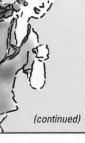

(continued)

What happens in respiratory acidosis *(continued)*

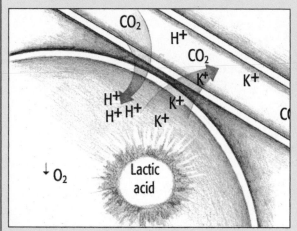

Step 6

As the concentration of H^+ overwhelms the body's compensatory mechanisms, the H^+ moves into the cells and K^+ moves out. A concurrent lack of O_2 causes an increase in the anaerobic production of lactic acid, which further skews the acid-base balance and critically depresses neurologic and cardiac functions. *Look for hyperkalemia, arrhythmias, increased $Paco_2$, decreased pH, and decreased LOC.*

Good job!

What causes it

- Neuromuscular problems
  - Guillain-Barré syndrome
  - Myasthenia gravis
  - Poliomyelitis
  - Spinal cord injury
- Respiratory center depression
  - Central nervous system (CNS) trauma
  - Brain lesions
  - Obesity
  - Primary hypoventilation
  - Use of certain drugs
- Lung diseases
  - Respiratory infections
  - Chronic obstructive pulmonary disease (COPD)
  - Acute asthma attacks
  - Chronic bronchitis
  - Acute respiratory distress syndrome
  - Pulmonary edema
  - Chest wall trauma
- Airway obstruction
  - Retained secretions
  - Tumors
  - Anaphylaxis
  - Laryngeal spasm
  - Lung diseases that alter alveolar ventilation

Trauma to the CNS and lesions are two causes of respiratory acidosis.

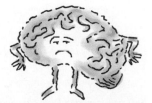

Drugs that can cause respiratory acidosis

Anesthetics
- Enflurane
- Halothane
- Isoflurane
- Nitrous oxide

Opioids
- Butorphanol
- Meperidine
- Morphine
- Nalbuphine

Sedatives and hypnotics
- Amobarbital
- Chloral hydrate
- Estazolam
- Flurazepam
- Lorazepam
- Pentobarbital
- Secobarbital
- Triazolam

What to look for

- Tachycardia
- Dyspnea with rapid, shallow respirations
- Nausea and vomiting
- Decreased deep tendon reflexes (DTRs)
- Warm, flushed skin
- Diaphoresis

Through the ages

Infants and acidosis

Infants commonly have problems with acid-base imbalances, particularly acidosis. Their low residual lung volume allows any change in respirations to alter their $Paco_2$, leading to acidosis. Their high metabolic rate yields large amounts of metabolic wastes and acids that must be excreted by the kidneys. Together with their immature buffer system, this leaves infants prone to acidosis.

- Restlessness
- Tremors
- Apprehension
- Confusion and decreasing level of consciousness (LOC)

What tests show

- Arterial blood gas (ABG) analysis
- Chest X-rays
  - Evidence of COPD
  - Evidence of pneumonia, pneumothorax, or other cause
- Electrolyte levels
  - Potassium level greater than 5 mEq/L (SI, 5 mmol/L)
- Other blood tests
  - Drug screening that may detect overdose

The ABCs of ABGs

This chart lists normal ABG levels for adult patients.

ABG	Normal level
pH	7.35 to 7.45
Paco$_2$	35 to 45 mm Hg
HCO$_3$$^-$	22 to 26 mEq/L

How it's treated

- Maintain a patent airway.
- Give a bronchodilator to open constricted airways.
- Administer supplemental oxygen (O$_2$) as needed.
- Expect to use a lower O$_2$ concentration for a patient with COPD. In such a patient, the medulla is accustomed to high

ABG results in respiratory acidosis

This chart shows typical ABG levels in uncompensated and compensated respiratory acidosis.

ABG	Uncompensated	Compensated
pH	< 7.35 (SI, < 7.35)	Normal
$Paco_2$	> 45 mm Hg (SI, > 5.3 kPa)	> 45 mm Hg (SI, > 5.3 kPa)
HCO_3^-	Normal	> 26 mEq/L (SI, > 26 mmol/L)

CO_2 levels, and a lack of O_2 stimulates breathing. Therefore, administering too much O_2 can diminish the stimulus to breathe and depress respiratory efforts.

- Give drugs to treat hyperkalemia.
- Give an antibiotic to treat infection.
- Perform chest physiotherapy to remove secretions from the lungs.
- Perform tracheal suctioning, incentive spirometry, and postural drainage, and assist with coughing and deep breathing as needed.
- Monitor for changes in the patient's cardiac rhythm and respiratory pattern.
- Closely observe the patient's neurologic status and report significant changes.
- Promote fluid intake and carefully track fluid intake and output.

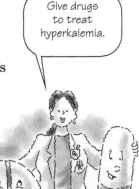

Give drugs to treat hyperkalemia.

Respiratory alkalosis

Key facts

- Respiratory alkalosis results from alveolar hyperventilation and hypocapnia.
- In respiratory alkalosis, pH is greater than 7.45 (SI, 7.45), and partial pressure of arterial carbon dioxide ($Paco_2$) is less than 35 mm Hg (SI, 4.7 kPa).
- Alkalosis may be acute, resulting from a sudden increase in ventilation, or chronic, which may be difficult to identify because of renal compensation.
- Any condition that increases the respiratory rate or depth can cause the lungs to eliminate too much CO_2. Because CO_2 is an acid, eliminating it decreases $Paco_2$ and increases pH.

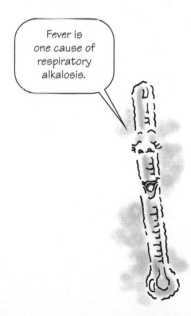

I see, I see

What happens in respiratory alkalosis

This series of illustrations shows how respiratory alkalosis develops at the cellular level.

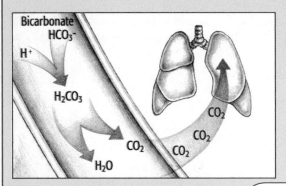

Step 1

When pulmonary ventilation increases above the amount needed to maintain normal CO_2 levels, excessive amounts of CO_2 are exhaled. This causes hypocapnia (a fall in $Paco_2$), which leads to a reduction in H_2CO_3 production, a loss of H^+ and HCO_3^- ions, and a subsequent rise in pH. *Look for a pH level greater than 7.45 (SI, 7.45), a $Paco_2$ level less than 35 mm Hg (SI, 4.7 kPa), and a HCO_3^- level less than 22 mEq/L (SI, 22 mmol/L).*

Follow the 6 steps to understand respiratory alkalosis.

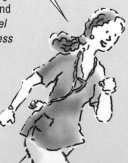

What happens in respiratory alkalosis *(continued)*

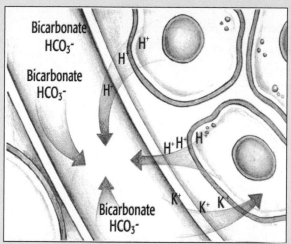

Step 2

In defense against the rising pH, H$^+$ is pulled out of the cells and into the blood in exchange for K$^+$. The H$^+$ entering the blood combines with HCO$_3^-$ ions to form H$_2$CO$_3$, which lowers pH. *Look for a further decrease in HCO$_3^-$ levels, a fall in pH, and a fall in serum K levels (hypokalemia).*

Look for a decrease in HCO$_3^-$ levels.

(continued)

What happens in respiratory alkalosis *(continued)*

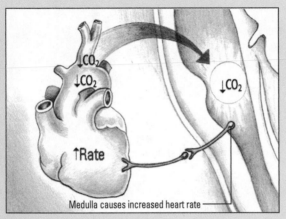

Medulla causes increased heart rate

Step 3
Hypocapnia stimulates the carotid and aortic bodies and the medulla, which causes an increase in heart rate without an increase in blood pressure. *Look for angina, ECG changes, restlessness, and anxiety.*

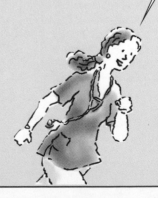

You're halfway there. Keep going!

What happens in respiratory alkalosis *(continued)*

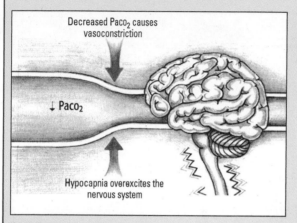

Decreased $Paco_2$ causes vasoconstriction

↓ $Paco_2$

Hypocapnia overexcites the nervous system

Step 4

Simultaneously, hypocapnia produces cerebral vasoconstriction, which prompts a reduction in cerebral blood flow. Hypocapnia also overexcites the medulla, pons, and other parts of the autonomic nervous system. *Look for increasing anxiety, diaphoresis, dyspnea, alternating periods of apnea and hyperventilation, dizziness, and tingling in the fingers or toes.*

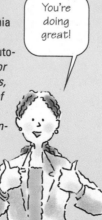

You're doing great!

(continued)

What happens in respiratory alkalosis (continued)

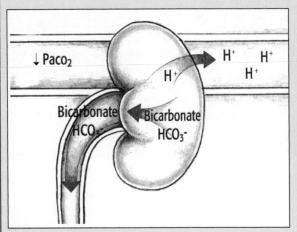

Step 5

When hypocapnia lasts more than 6 hours, the kidneys increase secretion of HCO_3^- and reduce excretion of H^+. Periods of apnea may result if the pH remains high and the $Paco_2$ remains low. *Look for slowing of the respiratory rate, hypoventilation, and Cheyne-Stokes respirations.*

What happens in respiratory alkalosis *(continued)*

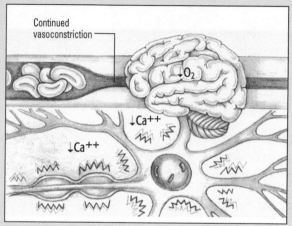

Step 6
Continued low Paco$_2$ increases cerebral and peripheral hypoxia from vasoconstriction. Severe alkalosis inhibits Ca^{++} ionization, which in turn causes increased nerve excitability and muscle contractions. Eventually, the alkalosis overwhelms the central nervous system and the heart. *Look for decreasing level of consciousness, hyperreflexia, carpopedal spasm, tetany, arrhythmias, seizures, and coma.*

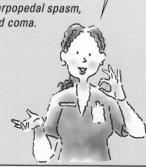

What causes it

- Hyperventilation
  - Pain
  - Anxiety
  - Salicylate intoxication
  - Use of certain drugs
- Hypermetabolic states
  - Fever
  - Liver failure
  - Sepsis
- Conditions that affect the respiratory control center
- Other causes
  - Acute hypoxia secondary to high altitude
  - Pulmonary disease
  - Severe anemia
  - Pulmonary embolus
  - Hypotension

Drugs that can cause respiratory alkalosis

Catecholamines
- Dobutamine
- Dopamine
- Epinephrine
- Isoproterenol
- Norepinephrine

Salicylates
- Aspirin
- Aspirin-containing compounds
- Diflunisal

Xanthines
- Aminophylline
- Oxtriphylline
- Theophylline

Other
- Nicotine

What to look for

- Tachycardia
- Syncope
- Dyspnea and increased respiratory rate and depth
- Diaphoresis
- Hyperreflexia
- Paresthesia

ABG results in respiratory alkalosis

This chart shows typical ABG levels in uncompensated and compensated respiratory alkalosis.

ABG	Uncompensated	Compensated
pH	> 7.45 (SI, > 7.45)	Normal
Paco$_2$	< 35 mm Hg (SI, < 4.7 kPa)	< 35 mm Hg (SI, < 4.7 kPa)
HCO$_3$⁻	Normal	< 22 mEq/L (SI, < 22 mmol/L)

- Tetany
- Anxiety
- Confusion
- Restlessness

What tests show

- ABG analysis
- ECG changes
  - Arrhythmias
  - Characteristic indications of hypokalemia or hypocalcemia
- Electrolyte levels
  - Serum calcium level below normal
  - Serum potassium level below normal
- Other blood tests
  - Toxicology screening with evidence of salicylate poisoning

How it's treated

- Correct the underlying cause, for example, by treating salicylate intoxication or sepsis.

- Administer supplemental O_2 if needed.
- Give a sedative if anxiety is the cause.
- Counteract hyperventilation by instructing the patient to breathe into a paper bag, which forces him to breathe exhaled CO_2 and raises the CO_2 level.
- If the cause is iatrogenic, adjust the ventilator settings.
- Monitor vital signs. Report changes in neurologic, neuromuscular, or cardiovascular functioning.
- Monitor ABG and serum electrolyte levels, and immediately report any changes.
- Institute seizure precautions as needed.

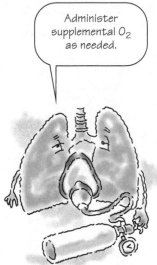

Metabolic acidosis

Key facts

- Metabolic acidosis is characterized by a pH level less than 7.35 (SI, 7.35) and an HCO_3^- level less than 22 mEq/L (SI, 22 mmol/L).
- Metabolic acidosis depresses the CNS and, if untreated, can lead to arrhythmias, coma, and cardiac arrest.
- Generally, metabolic acidosis is caused by HCO_3^- loss from extracellular fluid, metabolic acid accumulation, or both.

When I have a disorder it can cause metabolic acidosis.

I see, I see

What happens in metabolic acidosis

This series of illustrations shows how metabolic acidosis develops at the cellular level.

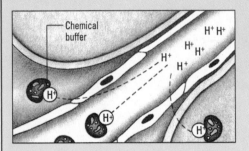

Step 1
As H^+ starts to accumulate in the body, chemical buffers (plasma HCO_3^- and proteins) in the cells and extracellular fluid bind with them. *No signs are detectable at this stage.*

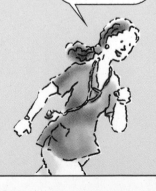

Follow the 6 steps to understand metabolic acidosis.

What happens in metabolic acidosis (continued)

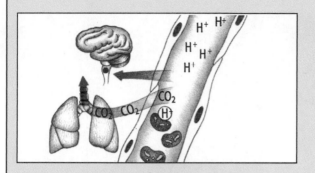

Step 2

If excess H^+ can't bind to the buffers, pH decreases, stimulating chemoreceptors in the medulla to increase the respiratory rate. The increased respiratory rate lowers the $Paco_2$, which allows more H^+ to bind with HCO_3^- ions. Respiratory compensation occurs within minutes but isn't sufficient to correct the imbalance. *Look for a pH level less than 7.35 (SI, 7.35), a HCO_3^- level less than 22 mEq/L (SI, 22 mmol/L), a decreasing $Paco_2$ level, and rapid, deeper respirations.*

> Look for a pH level less than 7.35.

(continued)

What happens in metabolic acidosis *(continued)*

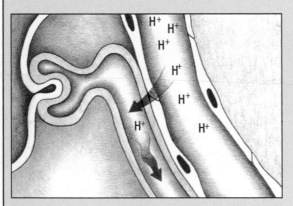

Step 3
Healthy kidneys try to compensate for acidosis by
secreting excess H+ into the renal tubules. Those
ions are buffered by phosphate or ammonia and
then are excreted into the urine in the form of a
weak acid. *Look for acidic urine.*

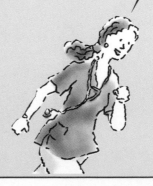

You're
halfway
there. Keep
going!

What happens in metabolic acidosis *(continued)*

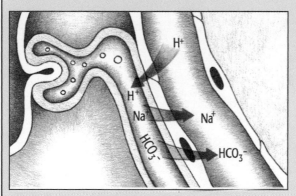

Step 4
Each time a H+ ion is secreted into the renal tubules, a
Na+ ion and a HCO₃⁻ ion are
absorbed from the tubules
and returned to the blood.
*Look for pH and HCO₃⁻
levels that return slowly
to normal.*

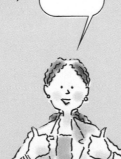

(continued)

What happens in metabolic acidosis *(continued)*

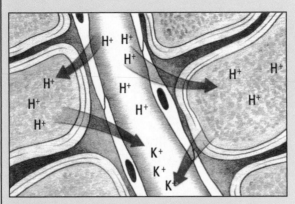

Step 5

Excess H+ in the extracellular fluid diffuses into cells. To maintain the balance of the charge across the membrane, the cells release K+ into the blood. *Look for signs and symptoms of hyperkalemia, including colic and diarrhea, weakness or flaccid paralysis, tingling and numbness in the extremities, bradycardia, a tall T wave, a prolonged PR interval, and a wide QRS complex.*

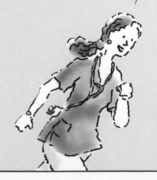

What happens in metabolic acidosis *(continued)*

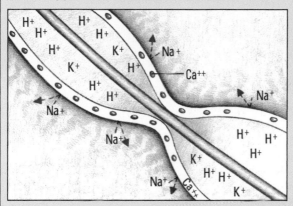

Step 6

Excess H^+ alters the normal balance of K^+, Na^+, and Ca^{++}, leading to reduced excitability of nerve cells. *Look for signs and symptoms of progressive central nervous system depression, including lethargy, dull headache, confusion, stupor, and coma.*

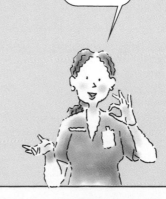

What causes it

- Ketone overproduction
  - Diabetes mellitus
  - Chronic alcoholism
  - Severe malnutrition
  - Starvation
  - Hyperthyroidism
  - Severe infection with fever
- Lactic acidosis
  - Shock
  - Heart failure
  - Pulmonary disease
  - Hepatic disorders
  - Seizures
  - Strenuous exercise
- Kidney disorders
  - Renal insufficiency
  - Renal failure with acute tubular necrosis
- GI disorders
  - Diarrhea
  - Intestinal malabsorption
  - Pancreatic or hepatic fistula
  - Urinary diversion to the ileum
  - Hyperaldosteronism

Drugs that can cause metabolic acidosis

Potassium-sparing diuretics
- Acetazolamide
- Amiloride
- Spironolactone
- Triamterene

Other drugs and substances (with poisoning or toxicity)
- Ammonium chloride
- Aspirin or other salicylates
- Ethylene glycol
- Hydrochloric acid
- Methanol

ABG results in metabolic acidosis

This chart shows typical ABG levels in uncompensated and compensated metabolic acidosis.

ABG	Uncompensated	Compensated
pH	< 7.35 (SI, < 7.35)	Normal
Paco₂	Normal	< 35 mm Hg (SI, < 4.7 kPa)
HCO₃⁻	< 22 mEq/L (SI, < 22 mmol/L)	< 22 mEq/L (SI, < 22 mmol/L)

What to look for

- Signs and symptoms of hyperkalemia
  - Abdominal cramps
  - Diarrhea
  - Muscle weakness
- Weakness
- Decreased DTRs
- Hypotension
- Warm, dry skin
- Lethargy
- Anorexia, nausea, and vomiting
- Confusion and decreasing LOC
- Dull headache
- Kussmaul's (rapid, deep) respirations

What tests show

- ABG analysis
- ECG changes characteristic of hyperkalemia
  - Tall T waves

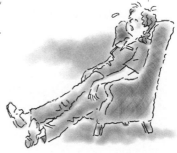

Lethargy is a sign of metabolic acidosis.

– Prolonged PR intervals
– Wide QRS complexes
• Electrolyte levels
  – Serum potassium level above normal
  – Increased anion gap (difference between the amount of sodium [Na] and HCO_3^- in the blood)
  – Plasma lactate level above normal in patients with lactic acidosis.
• Other blood tests
  – Blood glucose and serum ketone levels greater than normal in patients with diabetic ketoacidosis (DKA)

How it's treated

• Promote respiratory compensation, for example, by providing mechanical ventilation.
• Administer rapid-acting insulin to reverse DKA and move potassium back into the cells.
• Monitor the patient's potassium level.
• Administer sodium bicarbonate ($NaHCO_3^-$) I.V. to neutralize blood acidity if the patient's pH is less than 7.1 (SI, 7.1).
• Flush the I.V. line with normal saline solution before and after administering $NaHCO_3^-$ because the HCO_3^- may inactivate or cause precipitation of other drugs. Be aware that too much HCO_3^- can cause metabolic alkalosis and pulmonary edema.
• Begin dialysis for a patient with renal failure or a toxic drug reaction.
• If dopamine doesn't raise the blood pressure, check the patient's blood pH. A pH level less than 7.1 (SI, 7.1) causes resistance to vasopressors, such as dopamine. To make dopamine more effective, correct the patient's pH.
• Give an antidiarrheal if the HCO_3^- loss has been caused by diarrhea.
• Closely monitor the patient's neurologic status to detect changes in LOC and CNS deterioration.

Metabolic alkalosis

Key facts

- Metabolic alkalosis is characterized by a blood pH level greater than 7.45 (SI, 7.45) and a HCO_3^- level greater than 26 mEq/L (SI, 26 mmol/L).
- If untreated, this condition can lead to coma, arrhythmias, and death.
- Generally, metabolic alkalosis results from a loss of H^+ (acid), a gain of HCO_3^- ions, or both.

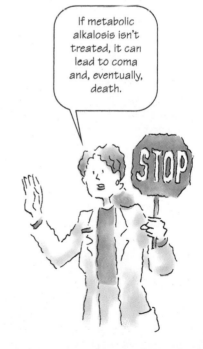

If metabolic alkalosis isn't treated, it can lead to coma and, eventually, death.

I see, I see

What happens in metabolic alkalosis

This series of illustrations shows how metabolic alkalosis develops at the cellular level.

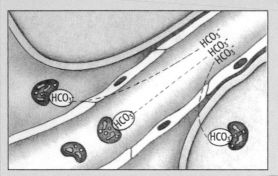

Step 1
As HCO_3^- ions start to accumulate in the body, chemical buffers (in extracellular fluid and cells) bind with the ions. *No signs are detectable at this stage.*

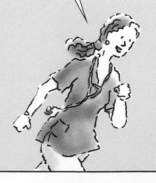

Follow the 6 steps to understand metabolic alkalosis.

What happens in metabolic alkalosis (continued)

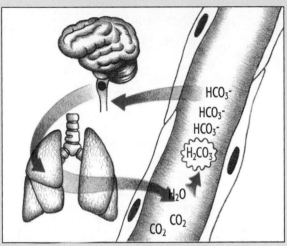

Step 2

Excess HCO_3^- ions that don't bind with chemical buffers elevate serum pH levels, which in turn depress chemoreceptors in the medulla. Depression of those chemoreceptors causes a decrease in respiratory rate, which increases the $Paco_2$. The additional CO_2 combines with H_2O to form H_2CO_3. *Note:* Lowered O_2 levels limit respiratory compensation. *Look for a serum pH level greater than 7.45 (SI, 7.45), a HCO_3^- level greater than 26 mEq/L (SI, 26 mmol/L), a rising $Paco_2$, and slow, shallow respirations.*

Look for slow, shallow respirations.

(continued)

What happens in metabolic alkalosis *(continued)*

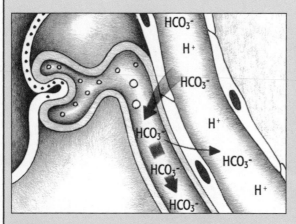

Step 3

When the HCO_3^- level exceeds 28 mEq/L (SI, 28 mmol/L), the renal glomeruli can no longer reabsorb excess HCO_3^-. That excess HCO_3^- is excreted in the urine; H^+ is retained. *Look for alkaline urine and pH and HCO_3^- levels that return slowly to normal.*

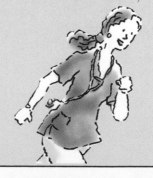

You're halfway there. Keep going!

What happens in metabolic alkalosis (continued)

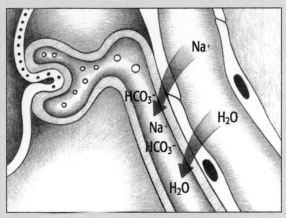

Step 4

To maintain electrochemical balance, the kidneys excrete excess Na^+, H_2O, and HCO_3^-. *Look for polyuria initially, then signs and symptoms of hypovolemia, including thirst and dry mucous membranes.*

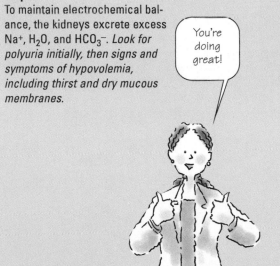

(continued)

What happens in metabolic alkalosis *(continued)*

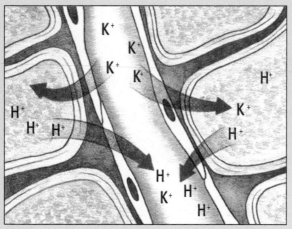

Step 5

Lowered H+ levels in the extracellular fluid cause the ions to diffuse out of the cells. To maintain the balance of charge across the cell membrane, extracellular K+ moves into the cells. *Look for signs and symptoms of hypokalemia, including anorexia, muscle weakness, and loss of reflexes.*

Only one more step to go!

What happens in metabolic alkalosis *(continued)*

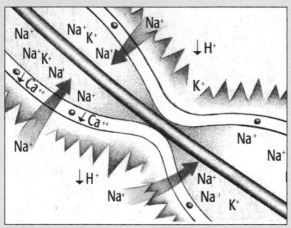

Step 6
As H+ levels decline, Ca++ ionization decreases. That decrease in ionization makes nerve cells more permeable to Na+. Na+ moving into nerve cells stimulates neural impulses and produces overexcitability of the peripheral and central nervous systems. *Look for tetany, belligerence, irritability, disorientation, and seizures.*

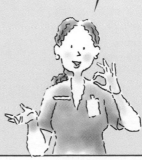

Good job!

What causes it

- Hypokalemia
  - Use of diuretics
  - Use of other drugs
- Excessive acid loss from the GI tract
  - Vomiting
  - Pyloric stenosis
  - Nasogastric (NG) suctioning
- Other causes
  - Cushing's disease
  - Overcorrection of acidosis
  - Kidney disease such as renal artery stenosis
  - Multiple transfusions

Drugs that can cause metabolic alkalosis

Antacids	**Loop diuretics**	**Thiazide diuretics**
• Calcium carbonate	• Bumetanide	• Chlorothiazide
• Sodium bicarbonate	• Ethacrynic acid	• Hydrochlorothiazide
	• Furosemide	

What to look for

- Hypotension
- Cyanosis
- Nausea and vomiting
- Anorexia
- Weakness
- Paresthesia
- Hyperactive reflexes
- Muscle twitching and tetany
- Polyuria
- Apathy and confusion

ABG results in metabolic alkalosis

This chart shows typical ABG levels in uncompensated and compensated metabolic alkalosis.

ABG	Uncompensated	Compensated
pH	> 7.45 (SI, > 7.45)	Normal
Paco$_2$	Normal	> 45 mm Hg (SI, > 5.3 kPa)
HCO$_3^-$	> 26 mEq/L (SI, > 26 mmol/L)	> 26 mEq/L (SI, > 26 mmol/L)

What tests show

- ABG analysis
- ECG
  - Low T waves that merge with P waves
- Electrolyte levels
  - Serum potassium, calcium, and chloride levels below normal

How it's treated

- For severe metabolic alkalosis, administer ammonium chloride I.V.
- Infuse 0.9% ammonium chloride no faster than 1 L over 4 hours. Faster administration can cause hemolysis of red blood cells. Don't give this drug to a patient with hepatic or renal disease.
- Discontinue thiazide diuretics and NG suctioning.
- Give an antiemetic to treat underlying nausea and vomiting.
- Give acetazolamide to increase renal excretion of HCO$_3^-$.
- Administer supplemental O$_2$, as needed, to correct hypoxemia.
- Institute seizure precautions as needed.

- Administer a diluted potassium solution using an infusion pump.
- Irrigate an NG tube with normal saline solution instead of tap water to prevent the loss of gastric electrolytes.
- Monitor the patient closely for muscle weakness, tetany, or decreased muscular activity.

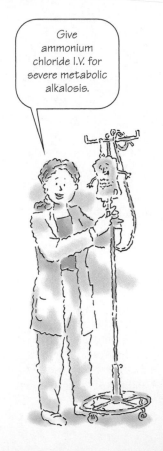

Give ammonium chloride I.V. for severe metabolic alkalosis.

Disorders that cause imbalances

5

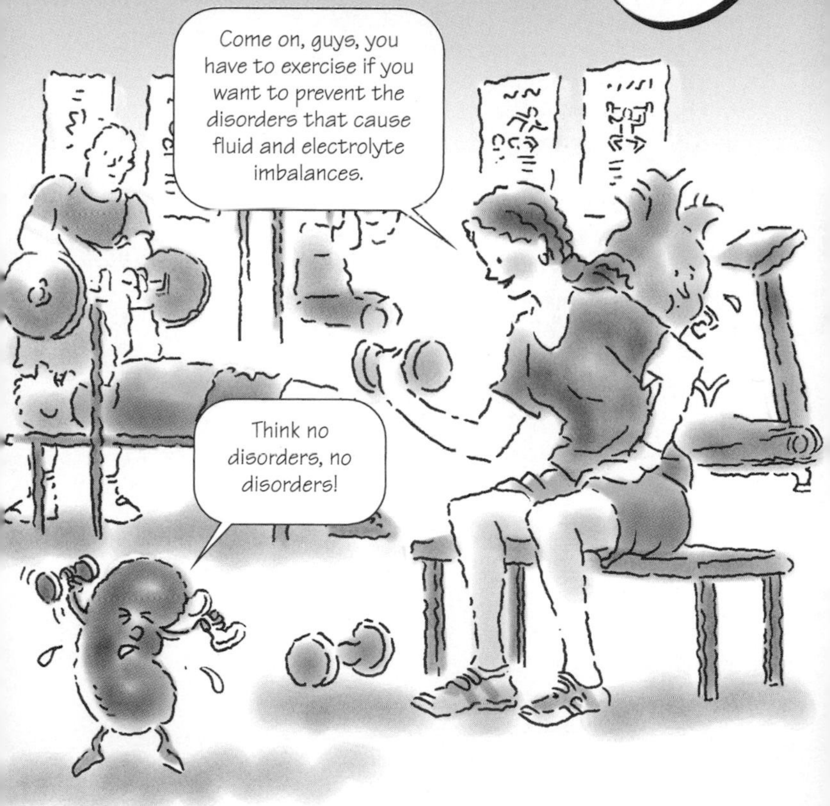

Heart failure

Key facts

- Heart failure is a syndrome of myocardial dysfunction that causes diminished cardiac output.
- Heart failure occurs when the heart can't pump enough blood to meet the body's metabolic needs.
- Any alteration in preload (volume), afterload (pressure), contractility (squeeze), or heart rate can decrease cardiac output and lead to heart failure.
- Normally, the pumping actions of the right and left sides of the heart complement each other, producing a synchronized and continuous blood flow.
- When a disorder occurs, one side of the heart may fail while the other continues to function normally for a time.
- If one side of the heart fails, the resulting strain eventually causes the other side to fail, resulting in total heart failure.
- Imbalances caused by heart failure include hypervolemia and hypovolemia, hyperkalemia and hypokalemia, hypochloremia, hypomagnesemia, hyponatremia, metabolic acidosis and alkalosis, and respiratory acidosis and alkalosis.

I didn't know failure was an option.

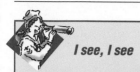

I see, I see

What happens in heart failure

Left-sided heart failure	Right-sided heart failure

| Left ventricular contractility diminishes. | Right ventricular contractility diminishes. |

| Left ventricle's ability to pump fails, producing increased heart rate, pale cool skin, arm and leg tingling, and arrhythmias. | Right ventricle's ability to pump fails, producing increased heart rate, cool skin, cyanosis, and arrhythmias. |

| Cardiac output to the body decreases. | Cardiac output to the lungs decreases. |

| Blood backs up into left atrium and lungs, causing dyspnea on exertion, confusion, dizziness, orthostatic hypotension, decreased peripheral pulses and pulse pressure, cyanosis, and S_3 gallop. | Blood backs up into right atrium and peripheral circulation, causing weight gain, peripheral edema, and engorgement of kidneys and other organs. |

Pulmonary congestion, dyspnea, and activity intolerance occur.

Pulmonary edema occurs.

Patient may develop right-sided failure if right ventricle becomes stressed from pumping against greater pulmonary resistance.

What causes it
- Myocardial infarction
- Myocardial fibrosis
- Ventricular overload
- Restricted ventricular diastolic filling

What to look for
Left-sided heart failure
- Third and fourth heart sounds
- Tachycardia
- Exertional dyspnea and paroxysmal nocturnal dyspnea
- Orthopnea and tachypnea
- Coughing, possibly with pink, frothy sputum
- Wheezes and crackles
- Oliguria
- Decreasing level of consciousness
- Fatigue
- Weakness

Right-sided heart failure
- Arrhythmias
- Chest tightness
- Jugular vein distention and rigidity
- Venous engorgement
- Palpitations
- Peripheral edema and ascites
- Cyanotic nail beds
- Anorexia and nausea
- Cool, clammy skin
- Cardiac arrest

What tests show
- Chest X-rays
  - Edema
  - Effusion
  - Congestion

- Echocardiograms
  - Enlarged heart chambers
  - Changes in ventricular function
- Electrocardiogram (ECG) tracings
  - Arrhythmias
- Hemodynamic pressure readings
  - Increased central venous pressure
  - Increased pulmonary artery wedge pressure

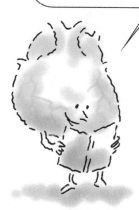

Wow! It says here that different conditions occur depending on which side of me fails.

How it's treated

- Place the patient in Fowler's position, and administer supplemental oxygen to ease his breathing and improve oxygenation.
- Give a diuretic to increase sodium and water elimination and reduce fluid overload.
- Monitor the patient carefully during diuretic therapy because diuretics can disturb the electrolyte balance and lead to metabolic alkalosis, metabolic acidosis, or other complications.
- Give an angiotensin-converting enzyme (ACE) inhibitor to decrease afterload and preload.
- To prevent hyperkalemia in a patient receiving a potassium-sparing diuretic, discontinue diuretic therapy before beginning ACE inhibitor therapy.
- Administer a beta-adrenergic blocker to decrease afterload and the heart's workload. Give a nitrate to dilate arterial smooth muscle.

- Give an inotropic drug, such as digoxin, to increase contractility and slow conduction through the atrioventricular node.
- Administer oral potassium in orange juice or with meals to promote absorption and prevent gastric irritation.
- Administer morphine to a patient with acute pulmonary edema.
- Prepare the patient with severe heart failure for surgery if needed. For example, an intra-aortic balloon counterpulsation or other assist device may be implanted, or heart transplantation may be needed when other treatment options aren't possible.
- Monitor the patient's sodium and fluid intake.
- Provide continuous cardiac monitoring during the acute and advanced stages of heart failure.

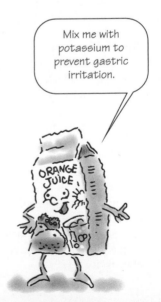

Respiratory failure

Key facts

- Acute respiratory failure results when the lungs can't sufficiently maintain arterial oxygenation or eliminate carbon dioxide (CO_2).
- If untreated, respiratory failure can lead to decreased oxygenation of the body tissues and fluid and electrolyte and acid-base imbalances.
- Causes of respiratory failure include disorders of the brain, lungs, muscles and nerves, and pulmonary circulation.
- In acute respiratory failure, impaired gas exchange can result from any combination of these factors: alveolar hypoventilation, ventilation-perfusion mismatch ($\dot{V}/\dot{Q}$), and intrapulmonary shunting.
- Imbalances caused by respiratory failure include hyperkalemia and hypokalemia, hypervolemia and hypovolemia, metabolic acidosis, and respiratory acidosis and alkalosis.

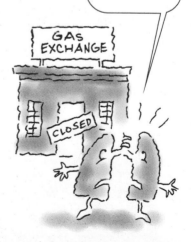

If gas exchange gets impaired, I could fail!

GAS EXCHANGE

CLOSED

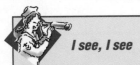

I see, I see

What happens in respiratory failure

Three major malfunctions account for impaired gas exchange and subsequent acute respiratory failure: alveolar hypoventilation, $\dot{V}/\dot{Q}$ mismatch, and intrapulmonary (right-to-left) shunting.

Alveolar hypoventilation

In alveolar hypoventilation (shown below as the result of airway obstruction), the amount of oxygen brought to the alveoli is diminished, which causes a drop in the PaO_2 and an increase in alveolar CO_2. The accumulation of CO_2 in the alveoli prevents diffusion of adequate amounts of CO_2 from the capillaries, which increases the $PaCO_2$.

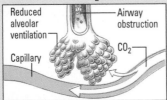

$\dot{V}/\dot{Q}$ mismatch

$\dot{V}/\dot{Q}$ mismatch, the leading cause of hypoxemia, occurs when insufficient ventilation exists with normal blood flow or when normal ventilation exists with insufficient blood flow. The PaO_2 is less than normal, but the $PaCO_2$ is normal because of normal ventilation in some parts of the lungs.

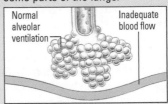

Intrapulmonary shunting

Intrapulmonary shunting occurs when blood passes from the right side of the heart to the left side without being oxygenated, as shown below. Shunting causes hypoxemia that doesn't respond to oxygen therapy.

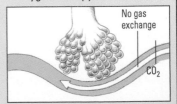

What causes it

- Conditions affecting the brain
  - Anesthesia
  - Cerebral hemorrhage
  - Cerebral tumor
  - Drug overdose
  - Head trauma
  - Skull fracture
- Lung disorders
  - Acute respiratory distress syndrome
  - Asthma
  - Chronic obstructive pulmonary disease (COPD)
  - Cystic fibrosis
  - Flail chest
  - Massive bilateral pneumonia
  - Sleep apnea
  - Tracheal obstruction
- Muscle and nerve disorders
  - Amyotrophic lateral sclerosis
  - Guillain-Barré syndrome
  - Multiple sclerosis
  - Muscular dystrophy
  - Myasthenia gravis
  - Polio
  - Spinal cord trauma
- Pulmonary circulation problems
  - Heart failure
  - Pulmonary edema
  - Pulmonary embolism

What to look for

- Increased heart rate
- Increased respiratory depth and rate
- Labored breathing with flared nostrils, pursed-lip exhalation, and the use of accessory breathing muscles

- Muscle retractions between the ribs, above the clavicles, and above the sternum
- Headache
- Anxiety and restlessness, progressing to confusion, agitation, and lethargy
- Cool, pale, clammy skin
- As respiratory failure worsens, be alert for arrhythmias, bradycardia, hypotension, cyanosis, dyspnea, diminished or absent breath sounds, wheezes, crackles, rhonchi, cardiac arrest, and respiratory arrest

> If you see signs of headache, anxiety, and cool, clammy skin, respiratory failure may be the cause of the imbalance.

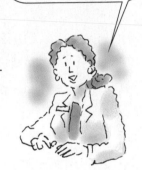

What tests show

- Chest X-rays
  – Evidence of a pulmonary disorder
- ECG tracings
  – Arrhythmias
- Arterial blood gas (ABG) analysis
  – Partial pressure of arterial oxygen (PaO_2) level less than 50 mm Hg (or less than 10 mm Hg in a patient with COPD)
  – Partial pressure of arterial carbon dioxide ($PaCO_2$) level greater than 50 mm Hg
  – pH less than 7.35 (SI, 7.35)
- Electrolyte levels
  – Serum potassium level greater or less than normal

How it's treated

- Administer supplemental oxygen in a controlled concentration, for example, by using a Venturi mask.
- Use caution when administering oxygen to a patient with COPD because an increased oxygen level can depress the breathing stimulus.

- If conservative treatment doesn't raise the oxygen saturation above 90%, intubate the patient, and provide mechanical ventilation.
- Avoid giving an opioid or a central nervous system (CNS) depressant to a patient who isn't mechanically ventilated because either drug may further suppress respirations.
- Give a bronchodilator to open the airways.
- Administer a corticosteroid, a diuretic, and an antibiotic, as prescribed.
- Perform chest physiotherapy and postural drainage, as needed, to promote adequate ventilation.
- Use suction if needed to clear the airways.
- Provide I.V. fluids to correct dehydration and to help thin secretions.
- Monitor and manage electrolyte and acid-base imbalances.
- Limit the patient's carbohydrate intake and increase his protein intake because carbohydrate metabolism causes more CO_2 production than protein metabolism.
- Position the patient for maximum lung expansion. Sit the conscious patient upright, as tolerated, in a supported, forward-leaning position.
- If the patient is retaining CO_2, encourage slow, deep breaths with pursed lips. Urge him to cough up secretions.

You'll want to make sure your patient's carbohydrate intake is limited.

Excessive GI fluid loss

Key facts

- Significant fluid loss from the GI tract is possible.
- If fluid isn't reabsorbed in the intestines, isotonic fluid loss occurs; if saliva is lost, hypotonic fluid loss occurs.
- Excessive fluids can be excreted as waste products or secreted from the intestinal wall into the intestinal lumen, resulting in fluid and electrolyte imbalances.
- Imbalances caused by excessive GI fluid loss include dehydration and hypovolemia, hypochloremia, hypokalemia, hypomagnesemia, hyponatremia, and metabolic acidosis and alkalosis.

> Fluid loss got you singing the blues? Read on and you'll be playing a happier tune.

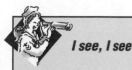

I see, I see

What happens in excessive GI fluid loss

GI fluid loss results from vomiting, suctioning, or altered GI motility.

Hypovolemia occurs.

To compensate, heart rate increases.

Tachycardia and hypotension occur as intravascular volume diminishes.

Body shunts blood to major organs, causing cool, dry skin.

Urine output and skin turgor decrease, and eyeballs appear sunken.

Electrolyte imbalances and arrhythmias cause weakness and confusion.

Patient's mental status deteriorates.

What causes it

- Physical removal of secretions
  - Vomiting
  - Suctioning
  - Increased or decreased GI tract motility
- Other causes
  - Anorexia nervosa or bulimia
  - Antibiotic use

– Bacterial infection
– Enema or laxative use
– Enteral tube feedings and ostomies
– Excessive intake of alcohol or illicit drugs
– Hepatitis or pancreatitis
– Poor absorption or digestion
– Pregnancy
– Pyloric stenosis in young children
– Young age

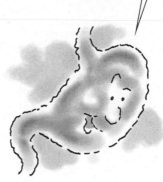

Poor digestion can lead to excessive GI fluid loss.

What to look for

- Decreased blood pressure
- Arrhythmias and tachycardia
- Increased heart rate
- Altered respirations
- Decreased urine output
- Decreased skin turgor and sunken eyeballs
- Cool, dry skin
- Confusion and weakness

Through the ages

Adolescents and excessive GI fluid loss

When treating an adolescent for excessive GI fluid loss, especially a female patient, assess for signs and symptoms of anorexia or bulimia. Teeth that appear yellow and worn away and a history of laxative or diet-pill use are two obvious signs.

Also, assess the patient for use of alternative diet therapies, particularly pills containing ma huang or ephedrine, which speed the metabolism by mimicking the effects of adrenaline on the GI system.

What tests show

- ABG analysis
  - Levels that reflect metabolic acidosis or alkalosis
- Electrolyte levels
  - Altered levels of certain electrolytes, notably potassium, magnesium, and sodium
- Other blood tests
  - Falsely elevated hematocrit (HCT)
- Other tests
  - Cultures of body fluid samples that identify the bacteria causing the infection

How it's treated

- Monitor for an increase in the amount of drainage from GI tubes, an increase in suctioning, or an increase in the frequency of vomiting or diarrhea.
- Assess the patient's fluid status by monitoring intake and output, daily weight, and skin turgor.
- Administer oral fluids that contain water and electrolytes, such as Gatorade or Pedialyte.
- Administer I.V. replacement fluids, using an infusion pump to prevent hypervolemia.
- If the patient is undergoing gastric suctioning, frequently check GI tube placement to prevent fluid aspiration.
- Irrigate the suction tube with isotonic normal saline solution.

Give your patient fluids containing water and electrolytes, such as Pedialyte.

- Never use plain water for irrigation. It draws more gastric secretions into the stomach in an attempt to make the fluid isotonic for absorption.
- When the patient is connected to gastric suction, restrict the amount of ice chips given by mouth because gastric suctioning of ice chips can deplete fluid and electrolytes from the stomach.
- Administer drugs, such as an antiemetic or antidiarrheal, to treat the underlying condition as prescribed.
- Evaluate serum electrolyte levels and pH.

Through the ages

Don't go too fast with fluids

Elderly patients can develop heart failure if I.V. fluids are infused too rapidly. Therefore, take caution when administering I.V. fluids to replace fluid losses in these patients.

Renal failure

Key facts

- Renal failure involves a disruption of normal kidney function and may be acute or chronic.
- Acute renal failure occurs suddenly and is commonly reversible. Chronic renal failure occurs slowly and is irreversible.
- Both types of renal failure affect renal function, producing imbalances as the kidneys lose the ability to excrete water, electrolytes, wastes, and acid-base products in urine.
- Causes of acute renal failure may be prerenal, intrarenal, or postrenal.
- Chronic renal failure develops in four stages: reduced renal reserve (glomerular filtration rate [GFR] 40 to 70 ml/min), renal insufficiency (GFR 20 to 40 ml/min), renal failure (GFR 10 to 20 ml/min), and end-stage renal disease (GFR less than 10 ml/min).
- Imbalances caused by renal failure include hyperkalemia, hypermagnesemia, hypernatremia and hyponatremia, hyperphosphatemia, hypervolemia and hypovolemia, hypocalcemia, and metabolic acidosis and alkalosis.

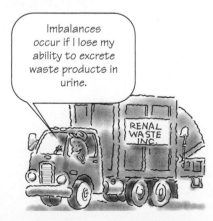

Imbalances occur if I lose my ability to excrete waste products in urine.

I see, I see

What happens in renal failure

Acute renal failure

Kidneys sustain damage, urine flow is obstructed, or renal blood flow diminishes.

▼

GFR decreases.

▼

Urine output falls to less than 400 ml in 24 hours.

▼

Kidneys fail.

▼

Nitrogenous waste products accumulate.

▼

BUN and serum creatinine levels rise.

▼

Uremia occurs.

▼

Uremia causes electrolyte imbalances, metabolic acidosis, and hypervolemia as renal dysfunction disrupts other body systems.

Chronic renal failure

Kidney function deteriorates gradually. Eventually, more than 75% of glomerular filtration is lost.

▼

Patient develops symptoms of uremia. Kidneys can no longer regulate fluid, electrolyte, and acid-base balance. Uremic toxins accumulate.

▼

Patient needs renal transplantation or dialysis.

What causes it

Acute renal failure

- Prerenal causes
  - Serious cardiovascular disorders
  - Hypovolemia
  - Peripheral vasodilation
  - Severe vasoconstriction
  - Renal vascular obstruction
  - Trauma
- Intrarenal causes
  - Acute tubular necrosis
  - Exposure to nephrotoxins or heavy metals
  - Aminoglycoside or nonsteroidal anti-inflammatory drug use
  - Ischemic damage from poorly treated renal failure
  - Eclampsia
  - Postpartum renal failure
  - Uterine hemorrhage
  - Crush injury
  - Myopathy
  - Sepsis
  - Transfusion reaction
  - Trauma
- Postrenal causes
  - Obstruction of the bladder, ureters, or urethra
  - Trauma

Chronic renal failure

  - Chronic glomerular disease
  - Chronic infection
  - Congenital anomaly
  - Vascular disease
  - Obstruction (as with calculi)
  - Collagen disease
  - Long-term nephrotoxic drug therapy
  - Endocrine disease

What to look for

Neurologic

- Burning, itching, and pain in the legs and feet
- Muscle irritability, twitching, and tremors
- Seizures
- Shortened attention span and memory
- Confusion
- Irritability
- Listlessness and somnolence
- Fatigue
- Coma
- Hiccups

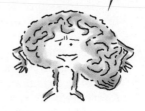

Hiccups can be a neurologic sign of renal failure.

Cardiovascular

- Arrhythmias
- Hypertension or hypotension
- Irregular pulse
- Tachycardia
- Pericardial rub
- Heart failure
- Anemia
- Weight gain with fluid retention

Pulmonary

- Dyspnea
- Crackles
- Decreased breath sounds, if pneumonia is present
- Kussmaul's respirations

GI

- Nausea and vomiting
- Metallic taste
- Dry mouth

- Inflammation and ulceration of GI mucosa
- Constipation or diarrhea
- Anorexia
- Bleeding
- Pain on abdominal palpation and percussion
- Ammonia breath odor

Integumentary

- Severe itching
- Loss of skin turgor
- Dry, scaly skin with ecchymoses, petechiae, and purpura
- Dry mucous membranes
- Dry, brittle hair that may change color or fall out easily
- Thin, brittle fingernails with lines
- Yellow-bronze skin color
- Uremic frost (in later stages)

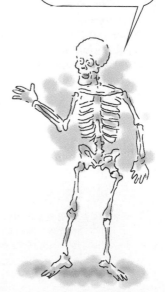

Pain in the bones and muscles may signal renal failure.

Genitourinary

- Anuria or oliguria
- Changes in urinary appearance or patterns
- Dilute urine with casts and crystals
- Amenorrhea in women
- Infertility
- Impotence in men
- Decreased libido

Musculoskeletal

- Muscle weakness
- Muscle cramps
- Bone and muscle pain
- Gait abnormalities
- Pathologic fractures
- Inability to ambulate

What tests show
- ABG analysis
  - Changes that indicate metabolic acidosis
  - Low pH
  - Low bicarbonate level
- ECG tracings
  - Tall, peaked T waves
  - Widened QRS complexes
  - Disappearing P waves, if hyperkalemia is present
- Electrolyte levels
  - Elevated potassium and phosphorus levels
- Other blood tests
  - Elevated blood urea nitrogen (BUN) and serum creatinine levels
  - Low HCT
  - Low hemoglobin (Hb) level
  - Mild thrombocytopenia
- Urinalysis
  - Casts
  - Cellular debris
  - Decreased specific gravity
  - Proteinuria

Through the ages

Age-related kidney changes

As people age, nephrons are lost and kidneys decrease in size. These physiologic changes decrease renal blood flow and may result in doubled BUN levels in older patients.

How it's treated

- Provide a low-protein, high-calorie diet and restrict the patient's intake of potassium, sodium, phosphorus, and fluid.
- Give a diuretic only if the patient has some degree of renal function.
- Monitor the patient's serum electrolyte and ABG levels. If imbalances occur, intervene appropriately.
- If the patient is anemic, administer iron and synthetic erythropoietin and provide blood transfusions as indicated.
- Administer a phosphorus-binding drug with meals to decrease the patient's phosphorus level.
- Monitor for ECG changes to help detect electrolyte imbalances.
- Monitor the patient's Hb level and HCT.
- Give sodium bicarbonate I.V., if needed, to control acute acidosis.
- Remember, sodium bicarbonate has a high sodium content and multiple doses may result in hypernatremia, which may contribute to the onset of heart failure and pulmonary edema.

Memory Jogger

To remember dietary changes needed to manage renal failure, think **"High, Lo, No."**

High calories

Low protein

No added salt (also watch the potassium)

- Begin dialysis to manage hypervolemia and electrolyte and acid-base imbalances. If the patient is hemodynamically unstable, provide continuous renal replacement therapy in the critical care setting.
- Frequently assess the hemodialysis access site for patency, bleeding, and signs of infection.
- Never use the arm with a hemodialysis graft or fistula for measuring blood pressure, drawing blood, or inserting I.V. catheters. Doing so could compromise the hemodialysis access site, which is the patient's connection for life-sustaining therapy.
- Check the route of excretion for drugs and adjust their dosages as needed.

Syndrome of inappropriate antidiuretic hormone

Key facts

- Syndrome of inappropriate antidiuretic hormone (SIADH) causes an excessive release of antidiuretic hormone (ADH) and disturbs fluid and electrolyte balance.
- ADH is released when the body doesn't need it. This results in water retention and sodium excretion.
- Imbalances caused by SIADH include hypervolemia and isovolumic hyponatremia.

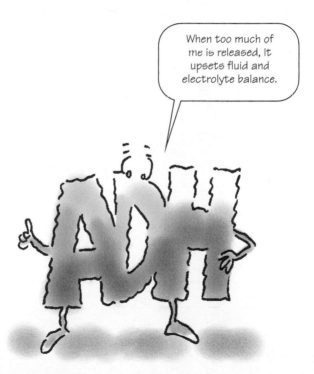

I see, I see

What happens in SIADH

The body secretes too much ADH.

▼

ADH increases renal tubule permeability.

▼

Increased tubule permeability increases water retention and extracellular fluid (ECF) volume.

▼

Increased ECF volume leads to:

▼ ▼ ▼ ▼

Reduced plasma osmolality	Dilutional hyponatremia	Diminished aldosterone secretion	Elevated GFR

▼ ▼

Sodium excretion increases, and fluid shifts into cells.		Patient develops thirst, dyspnea on exertion, vomiting, abdominal cramps, confusion, lethargy, and hyponatremia.	

What causes it
- Cancers
- CNS disorders
- Pulmonary disorders
- Use of certain drugs
  - Some oral antidiabetics
  - Chemotherapeutic drugs
  - Psychoactive drugs
  - Diuretics
  - Synthetic hormones
  - Barbiturates

What to look for
- Nausea and vomiting
- Anorexia
- Abdominal cramps
- Muscle twitching, tremors, and weakness
- Confusion
- Headache
- Lethargy
- Seizures, stupor, and coma

What tests show
- Electrolyte levels
  - Serum sodium level less than 135 mEq/L (SI, 135 mmol/L)
- Other blood tests
  - Elevated HCT and plasma protein levels
  - Serum osmolality less than 280 mOsm/kg
- Urine tests
  - Urine specific gravity above normal
  - Urine sodium level above 20 mEq/L (SI, 20 mmol/L)

How it's treated

- Restrict the patient's fluid intake to 500 to 1,000 ml/day.
- Consider a high-sodium, high-protein diet or urea supplements to enhance fluid excretion.
- Administer demeclocycline or lithium to block the renal response to ADH.
- Give a loop diuretic to prevent heart failure.
- Infuse a hypertonic saline solution to replace lost sodium.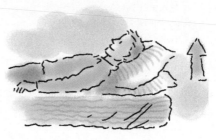
- Elevate the head of the bed to promote venous return. (Decreased venous return is a stimulus for ADH release.)
- Monitor the serum sodium level and adjust the flow rate of the I.V. saline infusion accordingly.
- A serum sodium level that rises too quickly puts the patient at risk for neurologic damage. Therefore, increase the serum sodium level by less than 12 mEq/L (SI, 12 mmol/L) in 24 hours.
- Correct the underlying cause of SIADH.

Burns

Key facts

- A burn interferes with the skin's ability to help keep out infectious organisms, maintain fluid balance, and regulate body temperature.
- Burns can result from thermal, mechanical, or electrical injuries as well as from exposure to chemicals or radiation.
- First-degree (partial-thickness) burns affect the superficial layer of the epidermis.
- Second-degree (deep partial-thickness) burns affect the epidermis and dermis.
- Third-degree (full-thickness) burns affect the epidermis, dermis, and underlying tissues.
- The extent of a burn can be estimated with a tool, such as the Rule of Nines or the Lund-Browder chart.
- Imbalances caused by burns include hyperkalemia and hypokalemia, hypernatremia and hyponatremia, hypervolemia and hypovolemia, hypocalcemia, metabolic acidosis, and respiratory acidosis.

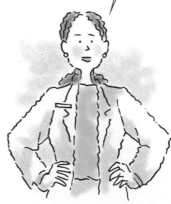

Burns make it difficult for the body to maintain fluid balance.

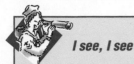

I see, I see

What happens in burns

Burn injury occurs.

▼

Capillary damage alters vessel permeability.
(Fluid accumulation phase begins.)

▼

Plasma escapes from intravascular space into interstitial space
(third-space shift). Blood becomes hemoconcentrated,
causing Hb and HCT to increase.

▼

Third-space shift leads to hypovolemia.

▼

Hypovolemia decreases cardiac output
and causes tachycardia and hypotension.

▼

Diminished kidney perfusion decreases urine output,
and the body releases aldosterone and ADH
as a result of stress and its response to burns.

▼

Aldosterone and ADH prompt kidneys to retain sodium and water,
and injured tissue releases acids,
which causes metabolic acidosis.

▼

Patient may develop fluid and electrolyte imbalances.

What causes it
- Thermal injuries
  - Exposure to dry heat (flames)
  - Exposure to moist heat (steam or hot liquids)
- Mechanical injuries
  - Friction or abrasion from skin rubbing harshly against a coarse surface
- Electrical injuries
  - Contact with high-voltage power lines
  - Immersion in water that has been electrified
  - Lightning strikes
- Chemical and radiation burns
  - Direct contact, ingestion, inhalation, or injection of acids, alkali, or vesicants

Fluid replacement formula

The Parkland formula is commonly used for calculating fluid replacement in burn patients. Vary volumes of infusions depending on the patient's response, especially his urine output.

Formula
4 ml of lactated Ringer's solution/kg of body weight/% of body surface area (BSA) over 24 hours.

Example
For a 68-kg person with 27% BSA burns:

4 ml × 68 kg × 27 = 7,344 ml over 24 hours.

Give ½ of the total over the first 8 hours after the burn and the remainder over the next 16 hours.

Estimating the extent of a burn

You can quickly estimate the extent of an *adult* patient's burns by using the Rule of Nines. This method divides an adult's body surface into percentages.

To use this method, match your adult patient's burns to the body chart shown here. Then add up the corresponding percentages for each burned section. The total — an estimate of the extent of your patient's burns — enters into the formula to determine his initial fluid replacement needs.

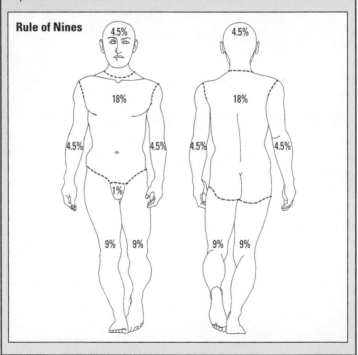

Rule of Nines

Estimating the extent of a burn *(continued)*

An infant's or child's body-surface percentages differ from those of an adult. For example, an infant's head accounts for a greater percentage of his total body surface when compared with an adult's. For an *infant* or *child,* use the Lund-Browder chart.

Lund-Browder chart

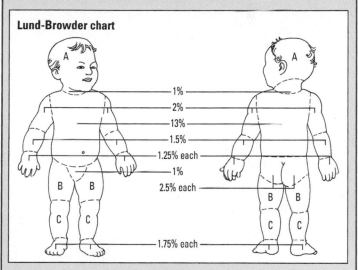

Relative percentages of areas affected by growth

At birth	1 to 4 yr	5 to 9 yr	10 to 14 yr	15 yr	Adult
A: Half of head					
9.5%	8.5%	6.5%	5.5%	4.5%	3.5%
B: Half of thigh					
2.75%	3.25%	4%	4.25%	4.5%	4.75%
C: Half of leg					
2.5%	2.5%	2.75%	3%	3.25%	3.5%

What to look for

First-degree burns
- Burns of the epidermis only
- Dry, painful wound
- Pink or red appearance
- Slight edema

Second-degree burns
- Burns of the epidermis and dermis
- Painful wound
- Swollen, red appearance
- Blisters
- Blanching and refill when pressure is applied
- Variable amount of scarring

Third-degree burns
- Burns of the epidermis, dermis, and tissues below the dermis
- Painless wound
- White to black (charred) color
- Dry, leathery appearance
- No blanching when pressure is applied

What tests show

- ABG analysis
  - Bicarbonate level below normal
  - pH below normal
- Electrolyte levels
  - Serum potassium level above normal
  - Serum sodium level below normal
- Other blood tests
  - BUN and creatinine levels above normal
  - Carboxyhemoglobin level above normal
  - Hb level and HCT above normal

- ECG tracings
  - Changes characteristic of electrolyte imbalances or my-ocardial damage
- Urine tests
  - Myoglobin in urine

How it's treated

Emergency burn care

- Extinguish any remaining flames on the patient's clothing.
- Don't directly touch the patient if he's still connected to live electricity. Unplug or disconnect the electrical source if possible.
- Assess the patient's airway, breathing, and circulation, and begin cardiopulmonary resuscitation, if needed.
- Assess the scope of the burns and other injuries.
- Remove the patient's clothing, but don't pull at clothing that sticks to the skin.
- Irrigate areas of chemical burns with lots of water.
- Remove from the patient jewelry or other metal objects that can retain heat and constrict movement.
- Cover the patient with a blanket.
- Send for emergency medical assistance.

Continuing burn care

- Treat severe facial burns or inhalation injuries with intubation, administration of high concentrations of oxygen, and positive-pressure ventilation.
- Provide initial fluid resuscitation with lactated Ringer's solution.
- Administer colloids, if prescribed, to increase blood volume.
- Use colloids cautiously in the immediate postburn period because they may worsen edema at the burn site.
- Infuse dextrose 5% in water to replace normal insensible water loss and losses caused by damage to the skin barrier. (If needed, add potassium to I.V. solutions 48 to 72 hours after the burn.)

- Insert a nasogastric tube to prevent gastric distention from paralytic ileus.
- Give an I.M. booster of tetanus toxoid.
- Avoid administering a prophylactic antibiotic because overuse of antibiotics fosters the development of resistant bacteria.
- Debride the wound. Assist with an escharotomy to prevent burn-induced compartment syndrome.
- Monitor for fluid, electrolyte, and acid-base imbalances.
- Give an analgesic 30 minutes before wound care. Use biological dressings for full-thickness burns and nonbiological dressings for partial-thickness burns.
- Maintain joint function with physical therapy and the use of splints and support garments.
- If bowel sounds are present, provide a diet high in potassium, protein, vitamins, fats, nitrogen, and calories. Provide enteral or parenteral nutrition if the patient can't tolerate oral intake.

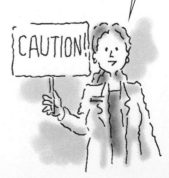

Treating imbalances

6

Treating fluid and electrolyte imbalances can be tricky.

You know, ma'am, if you break it, you buy it.

A look at treatments

- Depending on the type of imbalance and the patient's condition, treatment may require I.V. replacement therapy, total parenteral nutrition (TPN), dialysis, or transfusion of blood or blood products.
- Although each treatment corrects imbalances, it can lead to complications and requires expert clinical management.

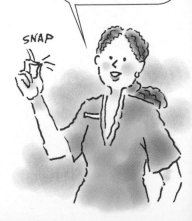

There are many different treatments that correct imbalances but after reading this chapter, it'll be a snap!

SNAP

I.V. replacement therapy

- Solutions for I.V. therapy fall into the broad categories of crystalloids (may be isotonic, hypertonic, or hypotonic) and colloids (always hypertonic).
- Crystalloids are solutions with small molecules that flow easily from the bloodstream into cells and tissues.
- Colloids are solutions with larger molecules used to expand plasma in patients who don't respond to crystalloids.
  - The effects of colloids may last several days.
  - Types include albumin, dextran, hetastarch, and plasma protein factor.
- I.V. replacement therapy provides the patient with life-sustaining fluids, electrolytes, and drugs.
- It allows for immediate and predictable therapeutic effects, the provision of fluid for a patient with GI malabsorption, and accurate I.V. drug titration.
- However, the patient may face drug and solution incompatibility, adverse reactions, or infection.

I.V. replacement therapy is a home run for patients in immediate need of fluids, electrolytes, and drugs.

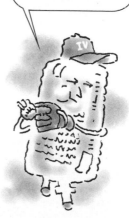

Isotonic solutions

Key facts

- Isotonic solutions have a concentration of dissolved particles (tonicity) equal to the intracellular fluid, so fluid doesn't shift between the extracellular and intracellular spaces.
- Their osmotic pressure is the same inside and outside cells.
- Cells neither shrink nor swell with isotonic fluid movement.
- Examples of isotonic solutions include dextrose 5% in water (D_5W), normal saline solution (0.9% sodium chloride), and lactated Ringer's solution.

Why it's done

D_5W

- To replace fluid loss and dehydration
- To treat hypernatremia

Normal saline solution

- To accompany blood transfusion
- To perform a fluid challenge
- To provide fluid replacement in patients with diabetic ketoacidosis (DKA)
- To treat hypercalcemia
- To treat hyponatremia
- To treat metabolic alkalosis
- To provide fluid resuscitation
- To treat shock

Lactated Ringer's solution

- To treat acute blood loss
- To treat burns
- To treat dehydration
- To treat hypovolemia caused by third-space shifting
- To treat lower GI tract fluid loss

What to consider

D₅W

- Remember, D_5W solution is initially isotonic and then becomes hypotonic when dextrose is metabolized.
- Use D_5W solution cautiously in patients with renal or cardiac disease because it can cause fluid overload.
- Don't use D_5W solution for resuscitation because it can cause hyperglycemia.
- D_5W doesn't provide enough daily calories for prolonged use and may eventually cause protein breakdown.

Normal saline solution

- Consider normal saline solution as a replacement for extracellular fluid (ECF).
- Don't use it in patients with heart failure, edema, or hypernatremia because it can lead to fluid overload.

Lactated Ringer's solution

- The electrolyte content of lactated Ringer's solution is similar to that of serum, but it doesn't contain magnesium.
- Because this solution contains potassium, don't use it in patients with renal failure; otherwise, hyperkalemia can occur.
- Don't use lactated Ringer's solution in liver disease because the patient can't metabolize the lactate.
- Don't use this solution in a patient whose pH is greater than 7.5 (SI, 7.5).

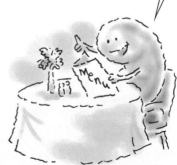

If I was failing, there's no way I'd order a lactated Ringer's solution.

Hypertonic solutions

Key facts

- Hypertonic solutions have greater tonicity than intracellular fluid.
- Their osmotic pressure is unequal inside and outside the cells.
- Hypertonic solutions draw water out of cells into ECF.
- Examples of hypertonic solutions include dextrose 5% in half-normal saline solution, dextrose 5% in normal saline solution, and dextrose 10% in water.

Why it's done

Dextrose 5% in half-normal saline solution

- To treat DKA after initial treatment with normal saline solution and half-normal saline solution
- To prevent hypoglycemia and cerebral edema in DKA treatment

Dextrose 5% in normal saline solution

- To treat addisonian crisis
- To treat hypotonic dehydration
- To treat syndrome of inappropriate antidiuretic hormone
- To provide a temporary treatment of circulatory insufficiency and shock if plasma expanders aren't available

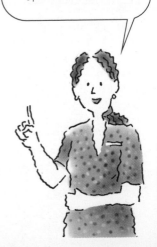

Dextrose 5% in normal saline solution is used to treat various imbalances such as hypotonic dehydration.

Dextrose 10% in water
- To treat conditions in which some nutrition with glucose is required
- To provide water replacement

What to consider

Dextrose 5% in half-normal saline solution
- In a patient with DKA, use this solution only when the glucose level falls below 250 mg/dl (SI, 13.9 mmol/L).

Dextrose 5% in normal saline solution
- Don't use this solution in cardiac or renal patients because of the danger of heart failure and pulmonary edema.

Dextrose 10% in water
- Monitor the patient's serum glucose level during therapy with dextrose 10% in water.

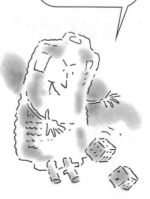

Don't roll the dice! Dextrose 5% in normal saline solution shouldn't be used in cardiac or renal patients.

Hypotonic solutions

Key facts

- Hypotonic solutions have less tonicity than intracellular fluid.
- Their osmotic pressure pulls water into cells from ECF.
- Cellular swelling results from hypotonic fluid therapy.
- An example of a hypotonic solution is half-normal saline solution (0.45% sodium chloride).

Why it's done

Half-normal saline solution

- To treat DKA after initial treatment with normal saline solution and before dextrose infusion
- To replace gastric fluid loss from nasogastric suctioning or vomiting
- To treat hypertonic dehydration
- To replace sodium and chloride depletion
- To provide water replacement

What to consider

Half-normal saline solution

- Use half-normal saline solution cautiously because it may cause cardiovascular collapse or increased intracranial pressure (ICP).
- Don't use this solution in a patient with liver disease, trauma, or burns.

Complications of I.V. therapy

- I.V. therapy requires careful patient monitoring and an ability to detect and properly deal with complications and flow issues.
- The most common complications of I.V. therapy are infiltration, infection, and phlebitis and thrombophlebitis.
- Other complications include extravasation, a severed catheter, an allergic reaction, an air embolism, speed shock, and fluid overload.

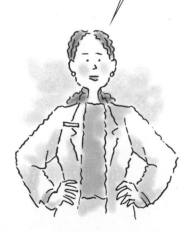

Remember to carefully monitor your patient while he's receiving I.V. therapy.

Infiltration

Key facts
- In infiltration, nonvesicant fluid leaks from the vein into surrounding tissue. This complication occurs when an I.V. access device becomes dislodged from a vein.

What to look for
- Pain, swelling, and leakage
- Coolness at the site
- Sluggish flow, even when a tourniquet is placed above the site
- Peripheral nerve damage (with a large infiltrate)

What to do
- Stop the infusion.
- Elevate the affected extremity.
- Remove the catheter and restart the infusion in another site in the other extremity.

How to prevent it
- Use the smallest catheter to accommodate the infusion.
- Avoid catheter placement in joint areas.
- Anchor the catheter.
- Consider using a gravity drip rather than an I.V. pump for a small I.V. catheter in a small vein.

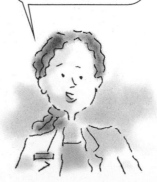

If infiltration occurs, remember three things: Stop the infusion, elevate the extremity, and restart the infusion at a different site.

Infection

Key facts
- Infection occurs because the puncture for venous access disrupts the integrity of the skin, the body's barrier to infection.

What to look for
- Drainage, tenderness, redness, and warmth at the I.V. site
- Hardness on palpation
- Fever and chills
- Elevated white blood cell (WBC) count

What to do
- Monitor the patient's vital signs and notify the doctor.
- Swab the site for culture and sensitivity testing.
- Remove the catheter as ordered.

How to prevent it
- Maintain sterile technique.
- Consider using a chlorhexidine antiseptic wipe or foam-impregnated disc for site care in a patient with a central line.
- Change catheter hubs routinely.
- Rotate peripheral I.V. catheter sites every 72 hours.

Phlebitis and thrombophlebitis

Key facts

- Phlebitis is an inflammation of the vein and can be mechanical, chemical, or bacterial.
- Thrombophlebitis is an irritation of the vein with clot formation.
- Phlebitis and thrombophlebitis can result from poor insertion technique, use of a solution or drug with an inappropriate pH or osmolality, or a peripheral I.V. catheter remaining in place too long.

What to look for

- Pain (more severe in thrombophlebitis), redness, swelling, or induration at the site
- Red line streaking along the vein
- Sluggish flow of the infusing solution
- Fever

> If you notice red line streaking along the vein, this may signal phlebitis or thrombophlebitis.

What to do

- Remove the I.V. line.
- Monitor the patient's vital signs and notify the doctor.
- Apply warm soaks to the site.

How to prevent it

- Choose large bore veins.
- Change the catheter every 72 hours when infusing a drug or solution with high osmolality.
- Treat a central line occlusion with a fibrinolytic.
- Flush the catheter exactly as directed by facility protocol.
- Dilute the drug and infuse at a slower rate.

Extravasation

Key facts
- Extravasation is the leakage of vesicant fluid into surrounding tissue.
- It results when drugs seep through veins and produce blistering and necrosis.

What to look for
- Discomfort, stinging, and burning at the infusion site (initially)
- Skin tightness, blanching, and lack of blood return
- Inflammation and pain (in 3 to 5 days)
- Ulcers and necrosis (in 2 weeks)

What to do
- Stop the infusion and notify the doctor.
- Infiltrate the site with an antidote as prescribed.
- Apply ice to the I.V. site initially, followed by warm soaks.
- Elevate the affected extremity.
- Assess circulation and nerve function of the affected extremity.

How to prevent it
- Follow facility policy when giving drugs that may extravasate.

Severed catheter

Key facts

- A severed catheter occurs when a piece of catheter becomes dislodged and is set free in the vein.
- It can result from defective equipment or poor insertion technique.
- A severed catheter is an extremely rare but serious complication.

What to look for

- Pain at the fragment site
- Weak, rapid pulses
- Cyanosis
- Decreased blood pressure
- Loss of consciousness

What to do

- Apply a tourniquet above the site of pain.
- Notify the doctor immediately.
- Monitor the patient.

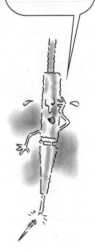

When I break, it's rare but serious.

How to prevent it

- Avoid reinserting a needle through its plastic catheter after the needle has been withdrawn.
- Pull peripherally inserted central catheter (PICC) lines out slowly, and never pull hard against resistance.

Allergic reaction

Key facts

- A patient may suffer an allergic reaction to a fluid, drug, I.V. catheter, or latex in the tubing.
- The source of the reaction may not be known.
- If left untreated, an allergic reaction may lead to anaphylaxis.

What to look for

- Red streak up the arm
- Rash and itching
- Watery eyes and nose
- Wheezing

What to do

- Stop the I.V. infusion immediately.
- Notify the doctor.
- Give supplemental oxygen and drugs, as prescribed.

How to prevent it

- Check the patient's record for allergies and hypersensitivity reactions.

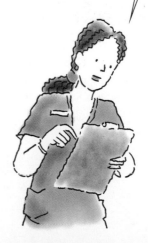

Always check and double check to ensure you're aware of allergies your patient may have.

Air embolism

Key facts
- An air embolism occurs when air enters the vein.
- This complication can result from inadvertent injection or infusion of an air bubble along with the fluid or drug.
- It's more likely to occur in central lines than in peripheral lines because central venous (CV) lines enter veins above the level of the heart.

What to look for
- Increased pulse rate
- Decreased blood pressure
- Respiratory distress
- Increased ICP
- Loss of consciousness

What to do
- Clamp the I.V. line.
- Notify the doctor immediately.
- Place the patient on his left side in Trendelenburg's position. This position allows air to enter the right atrium, where it can be removed more easily by the pulmonary artery.

How to prevent it
- Prime tubing completely.
- Tighten connections securely.
- Use an air detection device on the I.V. pump.

Speed shock

Key facts
- Speed shock is a systemic reaction that occurs when a substance is introduced into the circulation at a rapid rate.
- This complication commonly occurs when an I.V. solution or drug is given too quickly.

What to look for
- Decreased blood pressure
- Irregular pulse
- Facial flushing
- Severe headache
- Loss of consciousness and cardiac arrest

What to do
- Clamp the I.V. line immediately.
- Notify the doctor immediately.
- Provide supplemental oxygen.

How to prevent it
- Use an infusion control device.

Be a super hero and use an infusion control device to prevent speed shock.

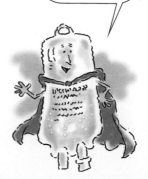

Fluid overload

Key facts
- Fluid overload can occur gradually or suddenly, depending on the patient's circulatory system and its ability to accommodate fluid.

What to look for
- Increased blood pressure
- Jugular vein distention
- Increased respirations
- Shortness of breath
- Crackles on auscultation
- Cough

What to do
- Slow the I.V. infusion rate.
- Notify the doctor and monitor the patient's vital signs.
- Keep the patient warm.
- Elevate the head of the bed.
- Give supplemental oxygen and drugs, as prescribed.

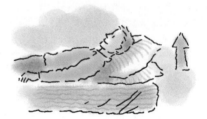

How to prevent it
- Always use an infusion pump to administer solutions.
- Always clamp the catheter when changing the I.V. solution.
- Consider the patient's size and age, and adjust fluid administration as needed.

TPN

- TPN is a highly concentrated, hypertonic nutrient solution administered by an infusion pump through a large central vein.
- It provides crucial calories, restores nitrogen balance, and replaces fluids, vitamins, electrolytes, minerals, and trace elements.
- Peripheral parenteral nutrition is a combination of lipids and amino acid-dextrose solution; it may be infused peripherally for less than 7 days.
- TPN is used to treat the following:
  – debilitating illness lasting longer than 2 weeks
  – a loss of 10% or more of pre-illness weight
  – a serum albumin level below 3.5 g/dl (SI, 35 g/L)
  – excessive nitrogen loss from a wound infection, fistula, or abscess
  – renal or hepatic failure
  – nonfunction of the GI tract lasting for 5 to 7 days

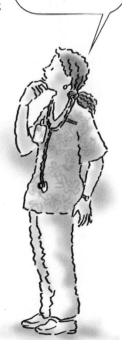

TPN provides calories; replaces fluids, vitamins, electrolytes, and minerals; and restores nitrogen balance. Now that's a pretty important treatment!

Common TPN additives

Key facts

- Such substances as electrolytes and vitamins are commonly added to TPN for specific purposes.
- Lipids may be added to TPN or infused separately.

Electrolytes

- Calcium promotes the development of bones and teeth and aids in blood clotting.
- Chloride regulates acid-base balance and maintains osmotic pressure.
- Magnesium helps the body absorb carbohydrates and protein.
- Phosphorus is essential for cell energy and calcium balance.
- Potassium is needed for cellular activity and cardiac function.
- Sodium helps control water distribution and maintains normal fluid balance.

OK, guys, are you ready to get to work?

Vitamins

- Folic acid is needed for deoxyribonucleic acid formation and promotes growth and development.
- Vitamin A is a fat-soluble vitamin that's necessary for cell and bone growth.
- Vitamin B complex helps the final absorption of carbohydrates and protein.
- Vitamin C aids in wound healing.
- Vitamin D is essential for bone metabolism and maintenance of the serum calcium level.

- Vitamin E is a fat-soluble vitamin that acts as an antioxidant to help protect cells from damage caused by the body's by-products of metabolism.
- Vitamin K helps prevent bleeding disorders.

Lipid emulsions

- Lipid emulsions supply patients with essential fatty acids and calories.
- These thick emulsions are usually given with TPN, but may be given alone via a peripheral or CV line.
- They assist in wound healing, RBC production, and prostaglandin synthesis.
- These emulsions shouldn't be given to patients with conditions that disrupt normal fat metabolism, such as pathologic hyperlipidemia, lipid nephrosis, and acute pancreatitis.
- Adverse reactions to lipid emulsions may be immediate (or early) or delayed (with prolonged administration).

Adverse reactions to lipid emulsions

Immediate reactions
- Back and chest pain
- Cyanosis
- Diaphoresis or flushing
- Dyspnea
- Headache
- Irritation at the site
- Lethargy or syncope
- Nausea and vomiting
- Thrombocytopenia

Delayed reactions
- Fatty liver syndrome
- Hepatomegaly
- Jaundice
- Splenomegaly

Other additives

- Acetate prevents metabolic acidosis.
- Amino acids provide the proteins needed for tissue repair.
- Micronutrients, such as zinc, chromium, selenium, and copper, help in wound healing and red blood cell (RBC) synthesis.
- Drugs, such as insulin, help manage hyperglycemia related to concentrated dextrose infusion.

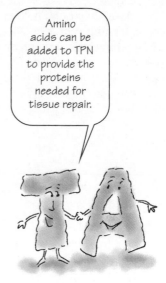

Amino acids can be added to TPN to provide the proteins needed for tissue repair.

Complications of TPN

Key facts

- Acid-base imbalances
- Electrolyte imbalances, with such effects as abdominal cramps, arrhythmias, confusion, lethargy, malaise, muscle weakness, seizures, and tetany
- Heart failure or pulmonary edema
- Hyperglycemia
- Hypoglycemia if insulin is added to the TPN solution
- Infection or sepsis
- I.V. cannula and CV catheter complications
- Liver dysfunction

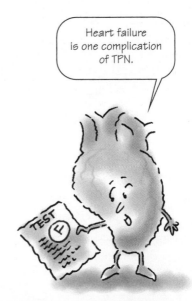

Heart failure is one complication of TPN.

Care related to TPN

Key facts

- Infuse TPN around the clock or for part of the day (usually at night), as prescribed.
- Use a silicone rubber (Silastic) catheter, which is preferred because it's more flexible and durable than other catheters and is compatible with many drugs and solutions.
- For therapy lasting 3 months or more, use a PICC line.
- Weigh the patient daily to assess his nutritional progress and to detect fluid overload. Also assess for edema, a sign of fluid overload.
- Monitor serum glucose level at least every 6 hours. Add insulin to the TPN solution, as prescribed.
- When TPN begins, monitor electrolyte and protein levels daily.
- Assess the patient's nitrogen balance with a 24-hour urine collection.
- Initiate TPN or a lipid emulsion slowly, and monitor for adverse reactions.
- With TPN, also monitor for signs and symptoms of hyperglycemia.
- Monitor for signs of refeeding syndrome, such as rapid decreases in the potassium, magnesium, and phosphorus levels.
- Don't use a TPN solution that's cloudy, has an oily layer, or contains particulate matter. Instead, notify the pharmacy.
- Also, don't allow a TPN solution to infuse for more than 24 hours.
- When discontinuing TPN, reduce the rate by 50% for 2 hours and then discontinue.

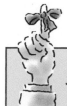

Memory jogger

To remember how to avoid the complication of refeeding syndrome when giving TPN to a severely malnourished patient, think, "Start low, and go slow."

Dialysis

- Dialysis is used to treat fluid and electrolyte imbalances when other treatments aren't effective in patients with acute or chronic renal failure.
- Hemodialysis and peritoneal dialysis are the most common renal replacement therapies used.
- Continuous renal replacement therapy (CRRT) is available for some hemodynamically unstable patients.
- Because dialysis filters out many drugs, such as antihypertensives and antibiotics, it should be performed before drug administration, not after.

> Dialysis isn't just skipping stones — it's used to treat imbalances when patients with acute or chronic renal failure haven't responded to other treatments.

Hemodialysis

Key facts

- Hemodialysis involves filtering the patient's blood outside the body through a semipermeable membrane that serves as an artificial kidney.
- This dialytic therapy requires access to the patient's circulation, a mechanism for transporting blood to and from the dialyzer, and a dialyzer that acts as a blood filter.

> Hemodialysis is used to rid a patient's blood of toxins.

The pros

- Effectively clears fluid and toxins from blood
- Requires no surgery because temporary vascular access can readily be established
- Offers a short treatment time (usually 4 hours)

The cons

- Can cause hemodynamic changes, which means it can't be used for hemodynamically unstable patients
- Produces adverse reactions, such as muscle cramping and complications of vascular access, such as clotting, infection, and bleeding
- Must be done three times per week
- Demands greater dietary and fluid restrictions than peritoneal dialysis does

I see, I see

Understanding hemodialysis

Hemodialysis is a process that filters the patient's blood outside of the body, as shown below. The blood passes through a dialyzer, which removes excess fluid and waste products. Then the blood is returned to the patient's circulation. A dialysate solution is used in this circuit to enhance the removal of waste products.

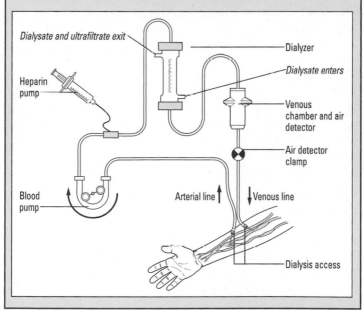

Peritoneal dialysis

Key facts

- Peritoneal dialysis involves using the peritoneal cavity as a filter.
- Through osmosis and diffusion, toxins move from the capillaries into dialysate solution (dextrose solution) instilled into the peritoneal cavity.
- The toxin-laden dialysate is then removed.

The pros

- Causes few hemodynamic complications
- Allows increased flexibility in the patient's lifestyle and schedule because patients can perform this therapy at home
- Allows more liberal fluid and dietary restrictions than hemodialysis does

The cons

- Can't be performed immediately after surgical placement of the peritoneal dialysis catheter, which requires 2 weeks of healing to prevent leakage
- Causes such complications as protein loss, bowel perforation, peritonitis, and hyperglycemia (from the dextrose solution)
- Isn't an option if the patient has extensive peritoneal adhesions from surgery

I see, I see

Understanding peritoneal dialysis

In peritoneal dialysis, the peritoneal cavity is used as a filter or natural dialyzer. In this continuous dialytic therapy, a dialysate (dextrose) solution is instilled into the peritoneal cavity through a peritoneal dialysis catheter, which extends from the abdominal wall into the peritoneal cavity, as shown here. At the end of the prescribed dwell time, the dialysate solution containing waste products and fluid is drained from the peritoneal cavity and immediately replaced by fresh dialysate solution.

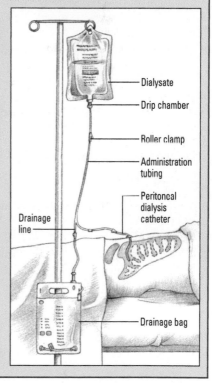

- Dialysate
- Drip chamber
- Roller clamp
- Administration tubing
- Peritoneal dialysis catheter
- Drainage line
- Drainage bag

CRRT

Key facts

- CRRT is used to manage fluid and electrolyte imbalances in hemodynamically unstable patients who can't tolerate hemodialysis.

The pros

- Allows immediate access to the patient's blood via a dual-lumen venous catheter
- Conserves cellular and protein components of blood
- Doesn't create dramatic changes in the patient's blood pressure, which commonly occurs with hemodialysis

The cons

- Must be performed by a specially trained critical care or nephrology nurse
- Must take place on an intensive care unit
- Requires CRRT equipment and supplies
- May pose issues of staff competency if CRRT is rarely used
- Is time-consuming

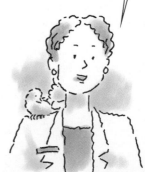

A little birdie told me that CRRT can only be performed by a nurse with special training.

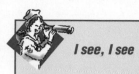

I see, I see

Following the CRRT circuit

In CRRT, a dual-lumen venous catheter provides access to the patient's blood. A pulsatile pump propels the blood through the tubing circuit.

The illustration here shows the standard setup for one type of CRRT called continuous venovenous hemofiltration. The patient's blood enters the hemofilter from a line connected to one lumen of the venous catheter, flows through the hemofilter, and returns to the patient through the second lumen of the catheter.

At the first pump, an anticoagulant may be added to the blood. A second pump moves dialysate through the hemofilter. A third pump adds replacement fluid if needed.

The ultrafiltrate (plasma water and toxins) removed from the blood drains into a collection bag.

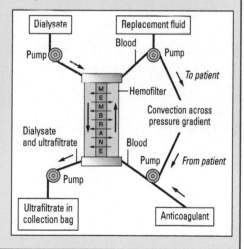

Transfusions

- Transfusions of blood and blood products can restore blood volume, correct deficiencies in the blood's oxygen-carrying capacity, and provide coagulation components.
- Depending on the blood product, different blood antigens (ABO blood group, Rh factor, and human leukocyte antigen [HLA] blood group) must be crossmatched to ensure compatibility between the donor and recipient's blood before transfusion.
- Transfusion therapy requires knowledge of the types of blood products, appropriate patient care, and techniques for handling transfusion reactions.

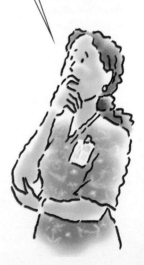

You must ensure compatibility before giving a transfusion.

Types of blood products

Key facts

- Blood products typically used for transfusions include whole blood, packed RBCs, granulocytes, fresh frozen plasma, cryoprecipitate, albumin, and platelets.
- The patient's own blood may also be stored and administered through a process called *autologous transfusion* (autotransfusion).

> Don't use whole blood if you're concerned about fluid overload.

Whole blood

- Whole blood is rarely used unless more than 25% of total blood volume is lost.
- It's available in 500-ml bags.
- It's used to treat hemorrhage, trauma, and major burns.
- Whole blood should be avoided if fluid overload is a concern.
- It requires lengthy storage, which may lead to hemolysis and hyperkalemia.
- It displays decreased RBC viability and function after 24 hours of storage.
- Whole blood requires ABO compatibility and Rh matching before administration.

Packed RBCs

- Packed RBCs are prepared by removing 90% of plasma around cells and adding an anticoagulant preservative.
- They're available in 250-ml bags.
- They reduce the risk of febrile, nonhemolytic reactions because about 70% of the leukocytes have been removed.
- Packed RBCs require ABO compatibility and Rh matching.

Granulocytes

- Granulocytes are also called WBCs.
- They're rarely used, except in patients with gram-negative sepsis or progressive soft-tissue infection that's unresponsive to antimicrobials.
- Granulocytes require Rh matching, preferably with HLA compatibility tests.

Fresh frozen plasma

- Fresh frozen plasma is prepared by separating plasma from RBCs and freezing it within 6 hours of collection.
- It contains plasma proteins, water, fibrinogen, some clotting factors, electrolytes, glucose, vitamins, minerals, hormones, and antibodies.
- It's used to treat hemorrhage, expand plasma volume, correct undetermined coagulation factor deficiencies, replace specific clotting factors, and correct factor deficiencies caused by liver disease.
- Fresh frozen plasma may require Rh matching, but not ABO compatibility testing.
- It may cause hypocalcemia when given in large volumes because the transfusion's citric acid binds with and depletes the patient's serum calcium.

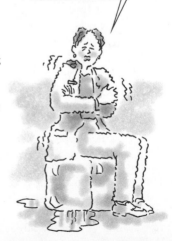

I know it's important to get the fresh plasma to a freezer, but this is ridiculous!

Cryoprecipitate

- Cryoprecipitate is also called *factor VIII*.
- It's the insoluble portion of plasma recovered from fresh frozen plasma.
- It's used to treat von Willebrand's disease, hypofibrinogenemia, factor VIII deficiency (antihemophilic factor), hemophilia A, and disseminated intravascular coagulation (DIC).
- Cryoprecipitate requires no ABO compatibility testing.

Albumin

- Albumin is extracted from plasma.
- It contains albumin, globulin, and other proteins.
- It's used to treat acute liver failure, burns, trauma, and hemolytic disease of the neonate.
- Albumin requires no ABO compatibility testing.

Platelets

- Platelets are primarily used to treat platelet dysfunction and thrombocytopenia.
- They're also used in patients who have had multiple transfusions of stored blood, acute leukemia, or bone marrow abnormalities.
- Platelets may require Rh matching.

Patient's own blood or blood components

- May be banked and used for autotransfusion.
- May require the patient to donate blood for a period of time (for elective surgery).
- May be withdrawn immediately before the procedure, replaced with I.V. fluid, and then reinfused after the procedure (for nonelective surgery and some elective surgery).
- May be used in a procedure that's expected to cause preoperative or intraoperative hemorrhage; shed blood is collected and then reinfused.

Care related to transfusions

Key facts

- Maintain sterile technique to protect the patient.
- Observe standard precautions to protect yourself. Wear a gown, gloves, and a face shield.
- Infuse blood products through an 18G or 20G I.V. catheter. Never use a smaller-gauge catheter or needle.
- Transfuse blood using a Y-type I.V. administration set (with filter), and infuse the blood over 2 to 4 hours.
- After starting the transfusion, remain with the patient and observe him carefully for the first 15 minutes.
- Be alert for acute adverse reactions, which typically occur within the first 15 minutes, but be aware that delayed reactions can occur up to 2 weeks later.
- Recheck vital signs 15 minutes after beginning the blood transfusion and again every hour.
- Use a pressure bag or a specialized infusion pump to administer a blood transfusion more rapidly if needed.

> Let's make sure that you and I agree on all of the details about your upcoming transfusion.

Pretransfusion safeguards

- Make sure the patient or his next of kin has signed an informed consent form.
- Explain the procedure to the patient.
- Because the religious beliefs of Jehovah's Witnesses preclude the use of blood products, make sure that refusal of blood reflects the pa-

tient's own decision and not coercion by family members or clergy. Consider consulting your facility's legal counsel on behalf of minors and adults incapable of giving their own consent.

- Review facility policy for administering blood.
- Assess the patient, documenting vital signs and other pertinent information. Notify the doctor if the patient has a fever of 100° F (37.8° C) or higher before the transfusion.

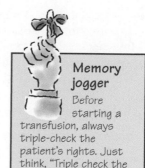

Memory jogger

Before starting a transfusion, always triple-check the patient's rights. Just think, "Triple check the two T's — right **transfusion** at the right **time**."

- Keep in mind the patient's other treatment needs. For example, if he's receiving an I.V. drug that can't be mixed with blood products, plan to insert another I.V. line.
- Check the orders for the type of transfusion to be given.
- Triple-check the patient's identity to make sure that the right patient receives the right transfusion at the right time.
- Ask the patient if he has ever had a transfusion reaction and, if so, under what conditions the transfusion was given and how it was resolved.

Flushing lines and using filters
- Flush lines with normal saline solution before and after infusing blood products.
- Also flush the I.V. line during the transfusion if the blood is dripping too slowly.
- Don't use a dextrose solution, which can cause hemolysis, or lactated Ringer's solution, which contains calcium and can clog the tubing.
- Filters work best when completely filled with blood.

- Use special filters if needed to trap leukocytes (leukocyte-depleting filters) or tiny clots and debris that can get through standard filters (microaggregate filters).
- When transfusing whole blood, reduce the risk of adverse reactions by adding a microfilter to trap platelets.

> Always check blood bags for leaks and clots.

Getting blood ready

- Obtain blood from the laboratory when you're ready to infuse it.
- Check the bag for leaks, discoloration, bubbles, and clots.
- Return questionable products to the blood bank.
- Don't store blood in a nursing-unit refrigerator because the temperature may be inaccurate and the blood could be damaged. If blood isn't refrigerated for 4 hours or more, it carries a high risk of bacterial contamination.
- Use a blood-warming device and special tubing if the order calls for blood to be warmed before administration such as when transfusing large quantities. Maintain the temperature between 89.6° and 98.6° F (32° and 37° C).

Giving platelets

- Transfuse platelets over 15 minutes.
- If the patient's history includes a platelet transfusion reaction, premedicate with an antipyretic or antihistamine, as prescribed.
- Avoid giving platelets when the patient is febrile.

- Check the platelet count 1 hour after the transfusion ends.

Giving other blood products
- Don't mix albumin with other solutions.
- Use albumin as a volume expander, if prescribed, until crossmatching for a whole blood transfusion is completed.
- Don't use albumin for patients with severe anemia, and give it cautiously to the patient with a cardiac or pulmonary disorder because heart failure may occur.

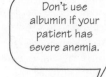

Don't use albumin if your patient has severe anemia.

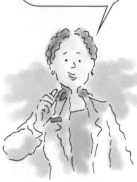

- Because cryoprecipitate's half-life is 8 to 10 hours, give repeated transfusions at those intervals to maintain a normal factor VIII level.
- Before granulocyte transfusion, premedicate the patient with diphenhydramine, if prescribed, and give an antipyretic for fever.
- Agitate the granulocyte container to prevent the cells from settling and unintentional delivery of a bolus infusion.
- Give a granulocyte transfusion with an antibiotic to treat infection, as prescribed, but don't give it with amphotericin B.

Providing posttransfusion care
- Continue to assess the patient as you remove the blood and tubing, and begin an infusion of normal saline solution to keep the vein open.
- Watch for signs of circulatory overload, especially in an elderly patient.
- Carefully monitor the infusion rate and I.V. site.

- Obtain laboratory tests, as ordered, to determine the effectiveness of the treatment.
- For an adult receiving 1 unit of packed RBCs, expect his hemoglobin level to increase by 1 g/dl (SI, 10 g/L) and his hematocrit to increase by 3%.
- For each unit of platelets infused, expect to see a rise of 5,000 to 10,000/mm^3 (SI, 5 to 10 X 10^9/L) in the platelet count.
- After giving clotting factors, expect to see an improvement in prothrombin time and partial thromboplastin time.
- Document blood product administration according to facility policy.

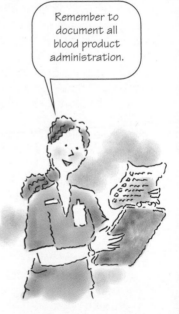

Transfusion reactions

- Transfusion reactions may be endogenous or exogenous.
- Endogenous reactions are caused by antigen-antibody reactions. These include allergic reactions, bacterial contamination, febrile reactions, hemolytic reactions, and plasma protein incompatibility.
- Exogenous reactions are caused by external factors in administered blood. These reactions include bleeding tendencies, circulatory overload, hypocalcemia, hypothermia, and potassium intoxication.

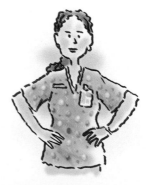

Transfusion reactions may be endogenous — caused by antigen-antibody reactions — or exogenous — caused by external factors.

Allergic reaction

Key facts
- An allergic reaction is caused by an allergen in donated blood. It may also be caused by donor blood that's hypersensitive to certain drugs.

What to look for
- Nausea
- Vomiting
- Fever
- Anaphylaxis (chills, facial swelling, laryngeal edema, pruritus, urticaria, and wheezing)

What to do
- Stop the infusion.
- Give antihistamines, as prescribed.
- Monitor vital signs and continue to assess the patient.
- Give epinephrine and corticosteroids, as prescribed.

> Don't gamble with allergic reactions. If your patient experiences nausea, vomiting, fever, or anaphylaxis, stop the infusion immediately.

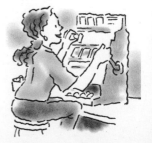

Bacterial contamination

Key facts
- Bacterial contamination is caused by organisms that survive the cold, such as *Pseudomonas* and *Staphylococcus* species.

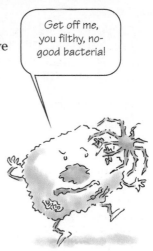

What to look for
- Diarrhea
- Abdominal cramping
- Vomiting
- Chills
- Fever
- Signs of renal failure
- Shock

What to do
- Stop the infusion.
- Give antibiotics, corticosteroids, and epinephrine, as prescribed.
- Maintain strict blood storage control.
- Change the administration set and filter every 4 hours or every 2 units.
- Infuse each unit of blood over 2 to 4 hours; stop the infusion if it lasts more than 4 hours.
- Maintain sterile technique.

Febrile reaction

Key facts

- A febrile reaction is caused by bacterial lipopolysaccharides.
- It occurs when the recipient's antileukocyte antibodies act against donor WBCs.

What to look for

- Increased pulse rate
- Palpitations
- Chest tightness
- Facial flushing
- Headache
- Cough
- Chills
- Fever up to 104° F (40° C)
- Flank pain

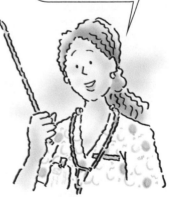

Chills, cough, flank pain, and chest tightness may indicate a febrile reaction.

What to do

- Stop the infusion.
- Administer antipyretics and antihistamines, as prescribed.
- If the patient needs further transfusions, use frozen RBCs and a leukocyte filter, and give acetaminophen as prescribed.

Hemolytic reaction

Key facts
- Hemolytic reaction is caused by ABO or Rh incompatibility.
- It may result from intra-donor incompatibility, improper crossmatching, or improperly stored blood.

What to look for
- Hypotension
- Chest pain and dyspnea
- Facial flushing
- Chills and fever
- Burning along the vein receiving blood
- Bloody oozing at the infusion site
- Flank pain
- Hemoglobinuria
- Oliguria followed by other signs of renal failure
- Shock

What to do
- Stop the infusion.
- Monitor the patient's vital signs, including pulse oximetry.
- Manage shock with I.V. fluids, oxygen, epinephrine, and vasopressors, as prescribed.
- Obtain a posttransfusion reaction blood sample and urine specimen for analysis.
- Observe for signs of hemorrhage from DIC.

Plasma protein incompatibility

Key facts
- Plasma protein incompatibility reaction is caused by immunoglobulin A incompatibility.

What to look for
- Hypotension
- Dyspnea
- Flushing
- Abdominal pain
- Diarrhea
- Chills
- Fever

What to do
- Stop the infusion.
- Administer oxygen, fluids, epinephrine, and corticosteroids, as prescribed.

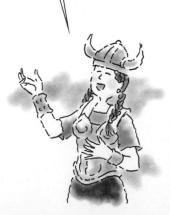

Watch out for plasma protein incompatablity — ee —e—EE—E— EEE...

Bleeding tendencies

Key facts

- Bleeding tendencies are caused by a low platelet count in stored blood.
- The low platelet count causes thrombocytopenia, which leads to bleeding.

What to look for

- Abnormal bleeding and oozing from cuts or breaks in the skin or gums
- Abnormal bruising
- Petechiae

What to do

- Give platelets, fresh frozen plasma, or cryoprecipitate, as prescribed.
- Monitor the patient's platelet count.

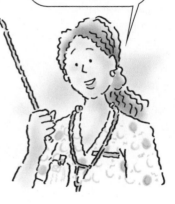

Abnormal bleeding from cuts on the gums and abnormal bruising are signs of bleeding tendency.

Circulatory overload

Key facts
- Infusing whole blood too rapidly may cause circulatory overload.

What to look for
- Hypertension
- Chest pain or tightness
- Increased CV pressure
- Jugular vein distention
- Flushed feeling
- Headache
- Dyspnea
- Back pain
- Chills and fever
- Increased plasma volume

What to do
- Slow or stop the infusion.
- Monitor the patient's vital signs.
- Use packed RBCs instead of whole blood.
- Give diuretics, as prescribed.

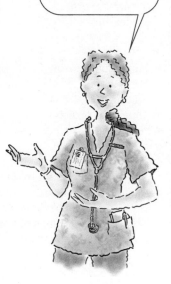

If whole blood is infused too rapidly, circulatory overload may occur.

Hypocalcemia

Key facts
- Hypocalcemia is caused by citrate toxicity.
- It occurs when citrate-treated blood is infused too rapidly and binds with calcium, causing a calcium deficiency.

What to look for
- Hypotension
- Arrhythmias
- Muscle cramps
- Nausea
- Vomiting
- Tingling in fingers
- Seizures

What to do
- Slow or stop the transfusion, if ordered. Expect a more severe reaction in a hypothermic patient or a patient with an elevated potassium level.
- Give calcium gluconate I.V. slowly, if prescribed.

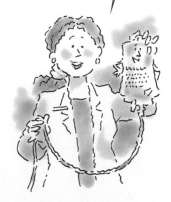

You may need to give I.V. calcium gluconate if your patient develops hypocalcemia from a transfusion.

Hypothermia

Key facts

- Hypothermia is caused by rapid infusion of large amounts of cold blood.
- It results in decreased body temperature.

What to look for

- Hypotension
- Arrhythmias, especially bradycardia
- Chills
- Shaking
- Cardiac arrest if core temperature falls below 86° F (30° C)

What to do

- Stop the transfusion.
- Warm the patient.
- Obtain an electrocardiogram (ECG) tracing.
- Warm the blood if the transfusion is resumed.

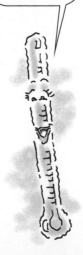

I get some pretty low numbers when hypothermia is involved.

Potassium intoxication

Key facts

- Potassium intoxication occurs with administration of stored plasma, which has an abnormally high potassium level.
- It's caused by hemolysis of RBCs.

What to look for

- Bradycardia
- ECG changes such as tall, peaked T waves
- Muscle twitching
- Flaccidity
- Diarrhea
- Intestinal colic
- Oliguria
- Signs of renal failure
- Cardiac arrest

What to do

- Stop the infusion.
- Obtain an ECG tracing and levels of glucose and such serum electrolytes as potassium.
- Give sodium polystyrene sulfonate, as prescribed.
- Give glucose 50% and insulin, bicarbonate, or calcium, as prescribed, to force potassium into cells.
- Give mannitol, and maintain vigorous hydration to encourage diuresis and prevent renal damage.

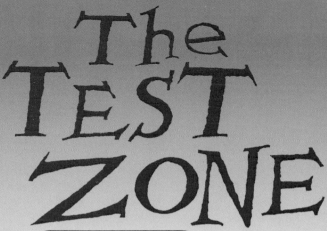

The TEST ZONE

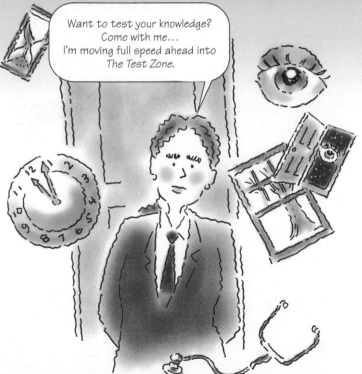

Want to test your knowledge?
Come with me…
I'm moving full speed ahead into
The Test Zone.

Chapter 1: Balancing basics

1. A patient has experienced an increase in blood pressure during a stress test. Which hormone helped bring his blood pressure back to normal?
  A. Renin
  B. Testosterone
  C. Aldosterone
  D. Progesterone

2. You're drawing blood from your patient for a sodium level. What types of electrolyte levels are measured?
  A. Intracellular
  B. Cellular
  C. Extracellular
  D. Intercellular

3. The ABG results for a 71-year-old patient who's in the intensive care unit are pH, 7.32; $Paco_2$, 47 mm Hg; HCO_3^-, 23. You interpret these results as:
  A. respiratory alkalosis.
  B. respiratory acidosis.
  C. metabolic alkalosis.
  D. metabolic acidosis.

4. A patient on your unit is hyperventilating. You can expect to see:
  A. Pao_2 of 70 mm Hg.
  B. Pao_2 of 110 mm Hg.
  C. Pao_2 of 95 mm Hg.
  D. Sao_2 of 95%.

Chapter 2: Fluid imbalances

5. A 91-year-old patient is admitted to your medical-surgical floor with confusion, dizziness, thirst, increased heart rate, decreased blood pressure, and a sodium level of 155 mEq/L. You suspect he has:
   A. hypovolemia.
   B. hypervolemia.
   C. dehydration.
   D. an acid-base imbalance.

6. A patient's X-ray shows pulmonary congestion; the doctor diagnoses pulmonary edema. What may have caused this condition?
   A. Loss of fluid
   B. Excess fluid volume
   C. Loss of sodium
   D. Low pulmonary hydrostatic pressure

7. A postoperative patient is being treated for hypovolemia. What should you do?
   A. Elevate the head of the bed.
   B. Give hypertonic solutions.
   C. Administer drugs to decrease blood pressure.
   D. Assess for crackles.

8. A nursing home patient has been admitted to the hospital with water intoxication. What will his admission orders most likely include?
   A. Monitor neurologic status.
   B. Administer a fluid challenge.
   C. Infuse hypotonic solutions.
   D. Use only tap water to irrigate NG tube.

Chapter 3: Electrolyte imbalances

9. A 75-year-old patient is admitted with agitation, confusion, intense thirst, and lethargy. His daughter tells you that he takes antacids with sodium bicarbonate many times a day. Which electrolyte imbalance should you suspect?
  A. Hyponatremia
  B. Hypokalemia
  C. Hypermagnesemia
  D. Hypernatremia

10. A 68-year-old patient is taking a beta-adrenergic blocker to treat his high blood pressure. His serum potassium level is 5.5 mEq/L. Which ECG changes would you expect to see?
  A. Shortened QRS complexes
  B. Tall, tented P waves
  C. Shortened PR intervals
  D. Tall, tented T waves

11. In an emergency, what would you administer to a patient with a high serum magnesium level?
  A. Magnesium sulfate
  B. Sodium polystyrene sulfonate (Kayexalate)
  C. Potassium chloride
  D. Calcium gluconate

12. Which electrolyte imbalance is relatively common; can lead to respiratory muscle paralysis, complete heart block, and coma; and can be the result of inadequate intake or inadequate absorption of the electrolyte?
  A. Hypophosphatemia
  B. Hypomagnesemia
  C. Hypokalemia
  D. Hyponatremia

Chapter 4: Acid-base imbalances

13. A 65-year-old woman who smokes two packs of cigarettes per day is hospitalized with pneumonia. She has tachycardia, is restless, and has dyspnea with rapid, shallow respirations. Her ABG results are pH, 7.29; $Paco_2$, 53 mm Hg; and HCO_3^-, 25 mEq/L. Which acid-base imbalance does this patient most likely have?
   A. Respiratory acidosis
   B. Respiratory alkalosis
   C. Metabolic acidosis
   D. Metabolic alkalosis

14. A patient who's on a ventilator has respiratory alkalosis. His pH is above normal and his $Paco_2$ is below normal. What electrolyte change should you monitor for?
   A. Serum potassium greater than normal
   B. Serum calcium greater than normal
   C. Serum sodium greater than normal
   D. Serum potassium less than normal

15. A 6-year-old girl comes to the emergency department with her mother, who's concerned about her lethargy and weakness. She says her daughter has recently lost a lot of weight but has a good appetite. She also frequently wakes up in the middle of the night to urinate. After blood levels are drawn, it's discovered that her pH is low, her HCO_3^- is low, and her blood glucose is elevated. Which acid-base imbalance does she have?
   A. Respiratory acidosis
   B. Respiratory alkalosis
   C. Metabolic acidosis
   D. Metabolic alkalosis

Chapter 5: Disorders that cause imbalances

16. A 68-year old patient has left-sided heart failure. What should you expect to see?
   A. Pulmonary congestion
   B. Peripheral edema
   C. Decreased cardiac output to the lungs
   D. Engorgement of the kidneys

17. One of your patients is in respiratory failure. What's true about the malfunctions that may have occurred?
   A. Alveolar hyperventilation is caused by airway obstruction.
   B. $\dot{V}/\dot{Q}$ mismatch occurs when normal ventilation exists with normal blood flow.
   C. Intrapulmonary shunting occurs when blood passes from the left side of the heart to the right side without being oxygenated.
   D. Alveolar hypoventilation occurs when the amount of oxygen brought to the alveoli is diminished.

18. A 41-year old patient is admitted to your unit. He hasn't been able to void for the past 24 hours, and he has some nausea and a dry, metallic taste in his mouth. He also has dyspnea. He's diagnosed with renal failure. What change will you expect to see?
   A. Serum potassium of 3.4 mEq/L
   B. Serum phosphorus of 4 mg/dl
   C. Tall, peaked T waves
   D. pH of 7.2

19. A 55-year old female with breast cancer is admitted with SIADH. Which intervention is appropriate for her condition?
   A. Keep the head of the bed lowered.
   B. Restrict fluid intake.
   C. Infuse D_5W.
   D. Give her a salt-free diet.

Chapter 6: Treating imbalances

20. Lactated Ringer's solution is ordered for a burn patient. What type of solution is lactated Ringer's solution?
- A. Isotonic
- B. Hypertonic
- C. Hypotonic
- D. Colloid

21. One of your patients has an order to have an I.V. started. What will you do to prevent infiltration?
- A. Use a large size catheter.
- B. Avoid placing the catheter in the antecubital space.
- C. Loosely tape the catheter in place.
- D. Always use an I.V. pump for a small I.V. catheter in a small vein.

22. A patient has been ordered TPN. What should you know about TPN therapy?
- A. TPN solution is usually cloudy.
- B. To discontinue TPN, just turn off and discard the remaining solution.
- C. During therapy, monitor for signs and symptoms of hyperglycemia.
- D. During therapy, monitor electrolyte and protein levels weekly.

23. A patient has been ordered to receive 1 unit of packed RBCs. What do you need to know before starting this procedure?
- A. You can flush the I.V. line during the transfusion with a dextrose solution or lactated Ringer's solution.
- B. After starting the transfusion, you must remain with the patient and observe him for 5 minutes.
- C. Infuse blood through an 18G or 20G I.V. catheter.
- D. Adverse reactions only occur within the first 15 minutes.

Answers

Chapter 1: Balancing basics

1. C. Aldosterone, produced as a result of the renin-angiotensin mechanism, helps maintain a balance of sodium and water and a healthy blood volume and pressure.

2. C. Only extracellular (serum) electrolyte levels are measured.

3. B. The patient's pH is low indicating acidosis, and his $Paco_2$ is high indicating respiratory acidosis.

4. A. A Pao_2 of 70 mm Hg represents hypoxemia and can cause hyperventilation.

Chapter 2: Fluid imbalances

5. C. Dehydration results when water loss isn't adequately replaced, which causes the listed signs and symptoms and laboratory values.

6. B. Excess fluid volume that lasts a long time can cause pulmonary edema. Fluid fills the alveoli and prevents the exchange of gases.

7. D. Monitor the patient for signs and symptoms of fluid overload, such as crackles, which may result from aggressive fluid replacement.

8. A. Water intoxication can cause changes in personality, behavior, and level of consciousness.

Chapter 3: Electrolyte imbalances

9. D. Antacids with sodium bicarbonate can cause hypernatremia.

10. D. ECG changes seen with hyperkalemia include tall, tented T waves and, possibly, a flattened P wave, prolonged PR intervals, widened QRS complexes, and depressed ST segments.

11. D. Calcium gluconate is a magnesium antagonist.

12. B. Hypomagnesemia can lead to respiratory muscle paralysis, complete heart block, and coma and can be the result of inadequate intake or inadequate absorption of magnesium.

Chapter 4: Acid-base imbalances

13. A. The patient's ABG analysis shows a pH level less than 7.35, a $PaCO_2$ level greater than 45 mm Hg, and a normal HCO_3^- level, which is consistent with respiratory acidosis.

14. D. During respiratory alkalosis, in defense against rising pH, hydrogen ions are pulled out of the cells and into the blood in exchange for potassium ions, causing a decrease in potassium levels.

15. C. The ketone overproduction that occurs with diabetes mellitus can cause metabolic acidosis.

Chapter 5: Disorders that cause imbalances

16. A. In left-sided heart failure, the left ventricle's ability to pump fails, cardiac output to the body decreases, and blood backs up to the left atrium and lungs causing pulmonary congestion and dyspnea.

17. D. In alveolar hypoventilation, the amount of oxygen brought to the alveoli is diminished, which causes a drop in PaO_2 and an increase in alveolar CO_2.

18. C. Diagnostic test results for a patient with renal failure will show ECG readings with tall, peaked T waves.

19. B. SIADH results in water retention and sodium excretion; therefore, you should restrict the patient's fluid intake to 500 to 1,000 ml/day.

Chapter 6: Treating imbalances

20. A. Lactated Ringer's solution is an isotonic solution that contains potassium. Isotonic solutions have a concentration of dissolved particles equal to the intracellular fluid, so fluid doesn't shift between the extracellular and intracellular spaces.

21. B. To prevent infiltration, avoid catheter placement in joint areas.

22. C. During TPN therapy, monitor the patient for signs and symptoms of hyperglycemia. Monitor blood glucose level at least every 6 hours and add insulin to TPN as prescribed.

23. C. Infuse blood products through an 18G or 20G I.V. catheter. Never use a smaller-gauge catheter or needle.

Scoring

☆☆☆ If you answered 21 to 23 questions correctly, great job! You're in a dimension all by yourself.

  ☆☆ If you answered 14 to 20 questions correctly, way to go! You're really in the zone.

    ☆ If you answered fewer than 14 questions correctly, review the chapters and try again! It won't be long until you see the light.

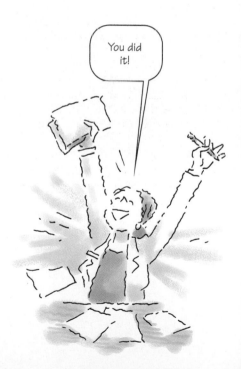

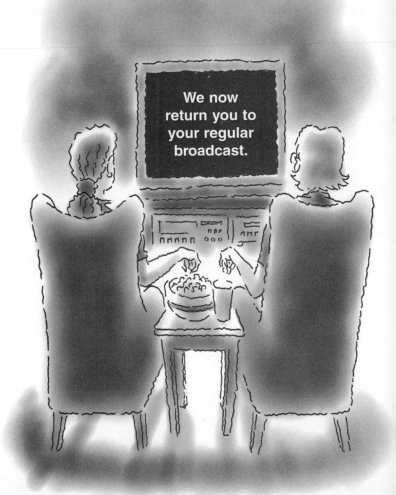

Selected references

Alexander, M., and Corrigan, A.M. *Core Curriculum for Infusion Nursing*, 3rd ed. Philadelphia: Lippincott Williams & Wilkins, 2003.

Becker, K.L., et al. *Principles and Practice of Endocrinology and Metabolism*, 3rd ed. Philadelphia: Lippincott Williams & Wilkins, 2003.

Bockenkamp, B., and Vyas, H. "Understanding and Managing Acute Fluid and Electrolyte Disturbances," *Current Practices* 13(7):520-28, 2003.

Cartotto, R., et al. "A Prospective Study on the Implications of a Base Deficit During Fluid Resuscitation," *Journal of Burn Care and Rehabilitation* 24(2):75-84, March-April 2003.

Critical Care Challenges: Disorders, Treatments, and Procedures. Philadelphia: Lippincott Williams & Wilkins, 2003.

Critical Care Nursing Made Incredibly Easy! Philadelphia: Lippincott Williams & Wilkins, 2004.

Fluid and Electrolytes Made Incredibly Easy!, 3rd ed. Philadelphia: Lippincott Williams & Wilkins, 2005.

Ignatavicius, D.D., and Workman, M.L. *Medical-Surgical Nursing: Critical Thinking for Collaborative Care*, 4th ed. Philadelphia: W.B. Saunders Co., 2002.

Johnson, R.J., and Feehally, J. *Comprehensive Clinical Nephrology*, 2nd ed. St. Louis: Mosby–Year Book Inc., 2003.

Morgera, S., et al. "Renal Replacement Therapy with High-Cutoff Hemofilters: Impact of Convection and Diffusion on Cytokine Clearances and Protein Status," *American Journal of Kidney Disease* 43(3):444-53, March 2004.

Nursing2005 Drug Handbook, 25th ed. Philadelphia: Lippincott Williams & Wilkins, 2004.

Smeltzer, S., and Bare, B. *Brunner & Suddarth's Textbook of Medical-Surgical Nursing*, 10th ed. Philadelphia: Lippincott Williams & Wilkins, 2004.

Swartz, R., et al. "Improving the Delivery of Continuous Renal Replacement Therapy Using Regional Citrate Anticoagulation," *Clinical Nephrology* 61(2):134-43, February 2004.

Teehan, G.S., et al. "Update on Dialytic Management of Acute Renal Failure," *Journal of Intensive Care Medicine* 18(3):130-38, May-June 2003.

Index

i refers to an illustration; t refers to a table.

i refers to an illustration; t refers to a table.

i refers to an illustration; t refers to a table.

i refers to an illustration; t refers to a table.